HEALTHCARE HANDBOOK

FOR SENIOR CITIZENS AND THEIR FAMILIES

KAREN MCGOUGH MONKS, MSN

ISBN: 1484964470
ISBN-13: 9781484964477

Library of Congress Control Number: 2013909467
CreateSpace Independent Publishing Platform
North Charleston, South Carolina

NOTICE

Healthcare is ever-changing. New research and healthcare experiences foster changes in therapy. Readers are advised to check with their primary care provider and/or pharmacist before making changes in their therapy or medications. This book aims to provide a handy reference to help guide senior citizens and family members to resources that can assist them when choosing appropriate healthcare services for themselves.

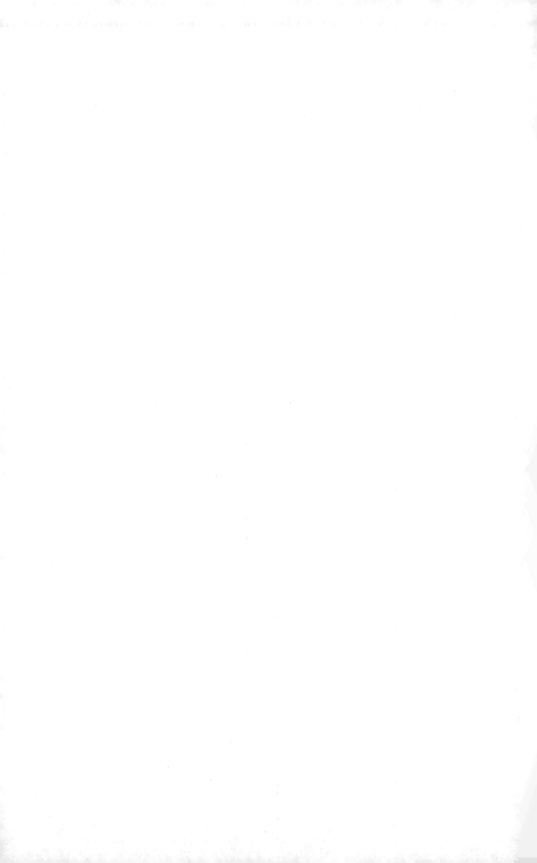

REVIEWERS

I want to express my appreciation to all of the following individuals who used their precious time to help review this book and provide valuable input:

Jennifer Breen M.S. CCC/SLP

Elaine Duemler BBA, ACS Volunteer

Betty Lundy MOA

Joseph Monks MBA

Laura Monks RN, BSN, RDH

Patrick Monks BS

Victoria Monks BA

Sandy Summers, RN, MSN, MPH

DEDICATED

To my family:

Patrick, my husband
Laura, my daughter
Joseph and Victoria, my son and
daughter-in-law
Keegan and Kylie, my grandchildren

For your support and encouragement.

GUIDELINES
FOR USING THIS BOOK

This book provides practical information about managing your healthcare decisions. It contains resources to assist seniors when choosing appropriate services for themselves. There are reminders throughout the book to emphasize important points.

This book contains information about:

- The various healthcare systems
- The roles of the different healthcare professionals
- How to stay healthy and safe
- Common Medical Conditions experienced by Seniors
- Different healthcare facilities and services
- Legal aspects related to healthcare
- End-of-life care
- Patient rights and responsibilities

It is suggested that you:

First: Read through the book to gain an overview of the content.

Next: Return to the sections that relate to your current healthcare situation, for closer review.

Lastly: Keep the book available to use as a resource when new healthcare issues occur.

TABLE OF CONTENTS

HEALTHCARE HANDBOOK FOR SENIORS AND THEIR FAMILIES

OR

How to Successfully Maneuver through the US Healthcare System(s)

CHAPTER I

INTRODUCTION

The discussions generated by the passage of the 2010 Healthcare Bill (Affordable Care Act) helped me realize there was a lack of understanding about the US healthcare system, by the general public. That realization helped me decide to write this handbook, which is intended to help senior citizens and their families better understand healthcare delivery, and help them learn how to maneuver through this Nation's healthcare system.

The term "**Healthcare System**" can be misleading. It makes it sound like it is a simple, one-dimensional organization, where in fact it is really a multifaceted system, which varies from State to State. A working knowledge of our system(s) will give everyone more control over their own healthcare.

FIFTY YEARS OF HEALTHCARE

Recently, I retired after 50 years as a registered nurse. During my career, I worked in many different areas of nursing and healthcare.

These areas included the hospital as a staff nurse, head nurse, and house supervisor; long term care as staff nurse and head nurse; home care as a case manager and staff educator; and nursing education as faculty and then director. I also spent 12 years on the board of directors for our community medical center. Additionally, I was an accreditation visitor for nursing programs, for several years.

All of these experiences provided me with a broad background in health care, including its various regulatory systems. I have also published two handbooks for healthcare professionals.

As expected, during those 50 years, my family and I needed to utilize various healthcare services, provided in this country. I appreciated the fact that, even with an intimate knowledge of the system, I still found it frustrating trying to utilize it. Frequently, I realized how fortunate I was that I knew my way around the networks. I often thought about how confusing it must be for someone who didn't have first hand knowledge of how to maneuver through the system.

FIFTY YEARS OF CHANGES

During the 50 years that I spent as a registered nurse, I have seen **remarkable changes** take place in healthcare. When I first started, the industry was much simpler than it is now. It is now so complicated that some people get lost in it. However, because of advances in healthcare in the past century, we are, also, able to live longer and have more productive lives, than we did 50 years ago.

As a nursing student in the **1950s,** I cared for patients with **polio,** who were kept alive in an iron lung. My classmates and I were some of the first groups of people to receive the Salk vaccine, for protection against Polio. Before the vaccine, our hospital reserved an entire nursing unit for the polio victims. The following year, there were only 3 or 4 polio patients at a time, on that same unit. The change was dramatic.

In the 1940s, **Penicillin** was just beginning to be used on a large scale. Before Penicillin and other antibiotics, healthcare workers were diligent about washing hands, and using other infection control measures. Then everyone became more lax, as antibiotics showed their magic.

As the years passed, we had to keep increasing the doses for antibiotics to remain effective. At first, we didn't realize that when we prepared antibiotic injections, droplets were inadvertently released into the hospital atmosphere, creating **super organisms,** such as MRSA (Methicillin-resistant Staphylococcus Aureus). Now we are back to using the tried and true infection control measures, like hand washing, that we used more faithfully before the discovery of Penicillin.

CPR (Cardiopulmonary Resuscitation) was developed and used by healthcare personnel in the **1960s.** We began teaching the general public how to perform CPR in the 1970s, which helped us keep people alive until we could get the victims to the hospital. If already in the hospital, we could keep the victim alive until the doctor got there. (Except for teaching hospitals, many healthcare facilities, especially in rural areas, did not have staff physicians available on site 24/7.)

These few examples demonstrate how we are able to save more lives today, and why there are more of us who are living longer and healthier.

NEW CHALLENGES

However (there is always a however), we are now facing different challenges in healthcare. We no longer worry about Polio, Diphtheria, or Small pox We are even doing better controlling cardiac conditions, and curing or controlling some cancers.

But we do have to be concerned about more **chronic conditions.** People still have strokes, although we are able to minimize the damage, if the victims get to the emergency room soon enough. People still develop **debilitating conditions,** such as Arthritis, COPD (chronic lung disease), Multiple Sclerosis, and Parkinson's Disease, just to name a few. **Diabetes** is a common condition, which is becoming more prevalent, with the increase of the incidence of obesity.

Probably the most feared conditions are the various **dementias,** such as Alzheimer's Disease. As we reach 65 years old and beyond, we will become more at risk for acquiring one of these conditions. There are things we can do to **maintain our health** and avoid losing our ability to function. There are, also, things we can do to **maximize our functioning,** even if we are faced with one of these conditions. I will address these issues more completely, later in this book.

In addition to my healthcare experience, I also have had personal experience advocating for my elderly cousin, Em (short for Esthermary). She was a lady who never married nor had any children. Her only sibling was killed in World War II, and her parents were deceased. She had been independent up until her middle 80s, when a young woman ran a red light and smashed her pickup truck into Em's car. As luck would have it, the young woman did not have auto insurance. Eventually, we were able to move Em into an assisted living facility, where she was able to remain relatively independent for 6 more years. Eventually, she appointed me as her Power of Attorney. I will discuss Em's situation as it applies, later in the book, especially the lessons we learned about available financial resources and legal issues that related to her healthcare.

Much of this book will deal with the various **healthcare organizations**, what **services** they offer, **regulations** they must follow, and how they can be **utilize**d. I have, frequently, realized that many people could use consultants to help them maneuver through the health care systems. Often, individuals are not aware of who and what services are available to them. Also, even if they did have that knowledge, they may not be able to afford to utilize them.

I will, also, **include** discussion about **common medical conditions** experienced by senior citizens. It is not practical to provide all medical answers in this book, but I will aim to provide **basic information,** along with helpful **resources.** Healthcare is continuously evolving, so I feel I can be most useful by **helping people learn where to find the information** that is needed.

HANDBOOK GOALS

My goal is to provide an **easy to use handbook,** to serve as a **resource** for average senior citizens and their families, to help make decisions about their healthcare. Additionally, this book is designed to help seniors access information to help discover what services are available, and how they might utilize these services.

There are many resources, one can use, to obtain healthcare information about specific issues. This book is designed to **organize this information in one place.** I will provide healthcare information, along with some reminders, to serve as a **ready reference** for its utilization. When you know the appropriate resources for health information, you will be better equipped to problem solve your particular health situation.

CHAPTER II

TYPES OF HEALTHCARE SYSTEMS

THIRD PARTY PAYERS

Probably the most frustrating aspect of healthcare is dealing with all of the different third party payers and their regulations. **Third party payers** are establishments **(third party)** which finance healthcare for the patient **(first party)** delivered by physicians, hospitals, or other healthcare providers **(second party).** Third party payers include public or governmental payers and private, such as insurance or charitable payers.

An aspect of healthcare, which contributes to increased frustration, is that the industry is always in a state of flux. Just when you think you understand the system, you find it is changing. This is one of the reasons why it is not easy to make corrections to the system. If changes are made in one area of healthcare, such as health insurance rules, you can expect a domino effect in other areas.

I always get nervous when our representatives in the government talk about making improvements in the healthcare system. Every time they do, there seems to be more paperwork required by the healthcare professionals. This requirement ends up with the providers spending more time recording information and less time for the patient.

When I first started working as a registered nurse, more than 50 years ago, nurses spent about 20 to 25% of their time doing paperwork. Now hospital nurses report that they spend about 50% of their time with paperwork or on the computer. That means 25 to 30% less time available for the patient. With the use of computerization, it is hoped that eventually, there will be less time documenting and more time for the patients. It is also hoped that computerization will provide increased safety in areas, such as medication administration.

Hospitals, clinics, doctor's offices, and other agencies that offer any kind of healthcare have had to add personnel, just to handle the complexities of billing. Billing used to just take someone with a business background, but now that person, also, needs to understand the coding involved with patient care and reimbursement, which involves a whole different area of expertise.

Obviously, all of this leads to increased healthcare costs. One problem is that, because most of us do not have to directly pay for all of our medical bills, many of us don't pay close attention to the bills, nor the cost of the services. However, the individual patient is in a better position to spot an inappropriate charge.

Part of the problem, when trying to correct certain discrepancies in healthcare, is there are several factors involved in each situation. To truly solve these problems, most of these factors need to be addressed. These factors not only involve all of the people and agencies who provide healthcare services, but also the people and agencies that receive the services. When we talk about correcting waste within the system, we need to not only look at the providers, but also those who receive the services.

Unfortunately, there will always be mistakes made, and there will always be some dishonest people, no matter how many regulations are in place. Hopefully, we can keep these at a minimum. You can help by paying attention to your bills and making sure they are consistent with the services you have received. Do not be afraid to ask questions if you do not understand something.

REMINDER: Always check your medical bills. Notice how much is charged for each service and how much is actually reimbursed.

In this chapter, I will describe the **major types of third party payers,** and some of their advantages and disadvantages. Having knowledge of these different systems and how they operate, should help you know what options are available when you are seeking healthcare services. I will also include resources and web sites, so you can seek additional information.

GOVERNMENT PROGRAMS

I will begin with Government run healthcare services. When I say Government, I am including national, state, and local governments.

MEDICARE and **MEDICAID** are probably the two most familiar government programs.

MEDICARE:

Signed into law in 1965, Medicare is administered by the **Centers for Medicare and Medicaid Services (CMS).** It is a part of the Department of Health and Human Services of the Federal Government.

This program is available to **three groups** of people. The group, with which most people are familiar, is American citizens **65 years or older.** Frequently, people get Medicare and Social Security eligibility confused. People can take early retirement with Social Security, but not be eligible for Medicare until they are 65 years old. There are some citizens who have not earned a sufficient number of quarters for coverage, through payment of payroll taxes, under the Federal Insurance Contributions Act (FICA). Those individuals may purchase Part A coverage, by contacting the Social Security office. The required amount of **quarters is 40,** which is earned by paying Medicare taxes for a **minimum of 10 years**.

Another category of Medicare eligible individuals is the **disabled.** In order for someone to be declared disabled for Medicare coverage, one **must be disabled for at least 24-29 months,** depending on whether they are already entitled to social security, or would be entitled if they had the required **QCs (quarters of coverage).** The intent is to be assured the individual is truly permanently disabled. As you can imagine, someone who has a sudden, devastating injury, such as a permanent spinal cord injury, will have a tough time for two years, before being eligible for some help. An **exception** to the 24 month wait, are individuals with **Amyotrophic Lateral Sclerosis (ALS).** Once they begin disability benefits, they can begin to receive Medicare Part B benefits.

The third category of Medicare eligible people is **End Stage Renal Disease (ESRD).** When I used to orient healthcare professionals for home care, I discovered most of them were not aware that this group of citizens were eligible for Medicare, even if they were not yet 65 years old. That made me wonder how many ESRD patients knew they were eligible.

ESRD is when the patient has **chronic kidney failure,** which is irreversible. When I first practiced as an RN, the kidney dialysis machine had just been developed. There were not many of them, available. I recall, at that time, each hospital had a 'Kidney Dialysis Committee,' that was charged with the task of deciding who could receive dialysis, and who could not. Usually, if you were over 65 years of age or had another chronic disease, you would probably not be eligible to receive the treatments.

As more dialysis treatments became available, it was observed that the people, who were being kept alive through dialysis, needed additional financial assistance. Many of them were not able to maintain full-time jobs, due to the amount of time required for their treatments. Frequently, they also had a variety of other medical complications.

Because of this, people with ESRD who require regular dialysis treatments, or a kidney transplant are, also, eligible for Social Security. This is the only chronic condition that qualifies people for these benefits, other than those conditions that are experienced by individuals who are 65 or older and the disabled.

If the individual, who is eligible for Medicare, already has full health insurance coverage, such as through their employment, that insurance remains the **primary insurance** and Medicare is the **secondary insurance.**

As many senior citizens realize, **Medicare Part A is not sufficient** to cover all of an elder's healthcare needs. One is wise to **sign up for Part B,** which is **cheaper, when first initiating Medicare** coverage. One can still enroll in Part B at any time, but it will cost more per month, if obtained after Medicare has been initiated.

REMINDER: It will cost you less, if you sign up for Medicare Part B **when you initiate** your Medicare Part A coverage.

Additionally, most elders find it necessary to have a secondary insurance (also called **Medigap**). **Part A** of Medicare mainly covers hospitalization, home care, and hospice services, whereas **Part B** covers outpatient services, such as outpatient surgery, physical and occupational therapy, and mental health care. It, **also, covers** outpatient laboratory services, kidney dialysis, and diabetic screening, training, and supplies.

I urge everyone to be sure to purchase **long-term care insurance.** Many people assume that Medicare covers long-term care, such as a stay at a skilled nursing facility (SNF). Medicare does cover some of the initial part of the stay at a SNF, as long as the patient demonstrates a skilled need, but it does not cover custodial care (bathing and feeding), if that is the only need. I will discuss this in more detail later, when discussing skilled nursing facilities.

REMINDER: A wise person will purchase Long Term Care insurance, if they can afford it. The sooner you purchase it, the less expensive it will be.

Medicare Part C is a another program called **Medicare Advantage** that can be used in lieu of using Parts A and B, and usually Part D. These are approved programs, such as HMOs (Health Maintenance Organizations) or PPOs (Preferred Provider Organizations). These two programs will be discussed in more detail later in this chapter.

Medicare Advantage programs must, at least, cover the same basic services, that are covered by Medicare, except for hospice care. Additionally, these programs may cover other services.

While you are enrolled in an advantage program, you are not eligible for Medicare. Actually, Medicare pays the Medicare Advantage company the monthly fee for your care. There are only certain times during the year when someone can join a Medicare Advantage program, or switch back to regular Medicare. The 2010 healthcare bill aims to improve the advantage programs by limiting the amount of money these companies can spend on administrative costs, and requiring all insurance companies to provide policy information to the consumer, in a uniform and clear manner.

REMINDER: It is important, that you notify all of your healthcare providers, when you switch third party payers, so they will be able to bill the proper payer. If they don't know you have switched, and bill the wrong entity, they will probably never receive reimbursement for their services. Frequently, the private insurance companies require pre-approval, before services can be rendered. If the provider does not find out that you have switched, before the services are provided, the payer will probably not pay for the service.

Medicare Part D helps cover the cost of **prescription medications**. This option is run by Medicare approved insurance companies. You are required to pay a monthly premium, and some plans require a yearly deductible. You, also, make a co-payment with each drug purchase. Presently, there is a **coverage gap,** with most drug plans. These plans help pay for the cost of an individual's drugs up to $2,830 for the year, then no longer pays until that individual's drug costs have reached $4,550. The **2010 Healthcare Bill** hopes to gradually close this gap, beginning in 2011. The goal is to provide complete drug coverage by 2020.

Individuals, who are **not eligible** for this program, and have difficulty paying for their medications, should **speak to their doctors** about this problem. The doctors may be able to order a drug that produces the same effects, but costs less, or they may have some samples they can provide. Also, some drug companies have programs, which the doctor can utilize to help with the cost of certain drugs, for patients in need.

REMINDER: Even if you do not need to pay for the full cost of the drug, pay attention to how much these medications cost. It will help remind you to follow the doctor's treatment regime, so you don't end up taking unnecessary medications.

MEDICAID:

Created in 1965, through Title XIX of the Social Security Act. The second major healthcare program, offered by the Federal Government, in conjunction with state governments. This program is **administered by the individual states,** and varies from state to state. It is intended for eligible **US citizens** and **legal resident aliens,** who live below a certain **income level,** and have limited resources. Another eligible group includes **individuals with certain disabilities.**

Included in the groups of eligible recipients are **some nursing home residents,** and **some disabled children** living at home. The term **"limited resources"** is used to describe adults who are eligible for Medicaid. This usually means that if an individual has a low income, but has other assets, such as savings or an IRA, **they must spend those savings down** before they become eligible.

Each state will have a specific level that savings must be below (i.e., $2,000 or below in most states). Usually, if the individual receives one or more annuity payments, they will not be eligible. **Do not assume** that, if your only income is Social Security, you are eligible for Medicaid. My cousin's monthly income from Social Security, was about

$200 more than the eligible level of income for Medicaid in our state.

However, **do not give up on exploring possibilities** for help. My cousin received two small annuity payments that did not help pay for her nursing home, but **disqualified** her for Medicaid. A social worker told me not to bother trying to get her qualified, but I tend to be persistent.

At first, I tried to cancel her annuities, and was basically told the only way she could cancel them was to die. I am sure when she first paid into those annuities in the 1950s, she thought the money would take care of her for life.

I then decided to call the local Medicaid office and was pleased to find they had a program for people like my cousin, to help her pay for her nursing home bills. Once she qualified for the program, she was required to pay for as much of her nursing home bill and medications her annuities and Social Security would cover; then the state paid for the rest of her care. She was allowed to keep a small stipend to use for personal needs.

REMINDER: Even if people say you are not eligible for a program, check it out for yourself. You may find that, although you do not qualify for one program, you may qualify for another one. Many states offer additional "state-only" programs to provide medical assistance for individuals, who do not qualify for Medicaid, but have a limited income.

Some people are **eligible for both** Medicare and Medicaid, such as those who are 65 years or older and have a qualifying low income. Medicaid will pay for their basic medical care and medications. Medicare will kick in when they require hospitalization or some type of skilled care.

Medicaid benefits **vary from state to state**. The federal government requires **certain basic coverage,** but each state can choose to provide additional services. Medicaid pays for, at least, part of the **medical bills** for those who are eligible. To obtain more specific information about what your particular state offers, you can go to **your state's web site.** If you do not have web access, you can begin by calling the **state's 800 number,** and request literature about their Medicaid program. Most communities will have a **local office,** that can give you more individualized information.

If you become a Medicaid recipient, you will be assigned a **case manager**. That person is available to answer questions and guide you through the process. Do not hesitate to call your case manager when you have a question. I found that my cousin's case manager responded to my inquiries in a very short period of time. **Be sure to thank them** for their help from time to time. They don't always receive much appreciation for their work.

Some states **contract with private companies** to provide the healthcare portion of their services. There is usually more than one company listed, from which you may choose. The state will usually provide some basic information about each company, to guide you. When you sign up with one of these companies, they will **also assign a case manager,** to help you with the healthcare part of your services. Having more than one case manager can be confusing when deciding to call about a problem. Their job is to help you, so don't hesitate calling someone. If you call the wrong person, they will let you know, and help you figure out who you should call.

When individuals initiate an application for Medicaid assistance, they are informed about the **"estate recovery" program**. Procedures to recover real property from the beneficiary's estate, in order to recover state money expended for services, are initiated after the beneficiary's death. The state is **required to remind** the recipients about the estate recovery program, on an annual basis.

Considerations are made to **prevent spousal impoverishment**. If one member of the couple is receiving care in a nursing facility, which can cost from $4,000-$6,000 per month, it doesn't take long for their resources to be drained. The state uses a formula to **calculate the spouse's share** of their resources, which can be legally protected. The maximum figure is readjusted from time to time. **Excluded** from the couple's resources, before the calculation is performed, are their home, household goods, one automobile, and burial funds.

After the **protected resource amount (PRA)** is determined, the remainder is considered available to go toward the cost of the care for the spouse in the nursing facility. Medicaid assistance for care can be used in long-term care facilities, home care, and community based services.

REMINDER: You can get more detailed information, about Medicare and Medicaid, by going to **www.medicare.gov,**

or Centers for Medicare and Medicaid Services (CMS) at **www.cms.gov.**

SOME OTHER programs provided by federal or state governments are Centers for Disease Control and Prevention (CDC), Indian Health Services, Federal Employees Health, Veterans Health Administration, Administration on Aging, Department of Health Services, and Department of Economic Security. Some people may find the need to utilize more than one of these agencies, at various times of their life.

CENTERS FOR DISEASE CONTROL AND PREVENTION (CDC):

The CDC was established in 1946, as the Communicable Disease Center. Today, the CDC is concerned with the **public health of the nation.** It aims to promote health, and prevent and control infection, disease, and injuries. It, also, provides preparedness for environmental and health threats (including bioterrorism), and responds to health emergencies. It works with state health departments and other agencies to provide systematic health surveillance.

The **State Health Departments** cooperate with CDC to investigate, prevent, and respond to **disease outbreaks,** implement strategies to **prevent diseases**, plan for and respond to **public health emergencies,** and maintain **health statistics**. They provide programs, for all members of the community, that **promote health** through nutrition, child care, and health promotion. They provide **services** for well baby clinics and immunizations for children and

19

adults, as well as communicable disease control, such as for tuberculosis and sexually transmitted diseases.

INDIAN HEALTH SERVICES (IHS):

IHS provides healthcare services to **Native Americans,** including Alaskan Natives. These services involve 33 hospitals, 59 health centers, and 50 health stations. The department was first established in 1787 under the Bureau of Indian Affairs, and later in 1955, was moved to IHS.

These healthcare services are provided for any **registered Indian/Alaskan Native,** regardless of tribe or income. IHS provides these healthcare services, either through its hospitals or clinics, or through tribal contracts. The services, provided on a particular reservation, are designated for their own tribal members first. Other Native Americans can receive care there, only if space is available, after the local tribe has received care. Native Americans. who leave their tribal homes, can apply for low income healthcare in the general community, including access to Medicaid.

FEDERAL EMPLOYEES HEALTH BENEFITS PROGRAM (FEHBP):

FEHBP was created, in 1960, for all federal employees and their dependents, including members of the US Congress. At first, the intent was to have a single plan, controlled by the federal government, but there were so many different groups involved, each had their own idea of the type of plan they needed. As a result, it ended up being a system of many competitive health plans.

Employees can choose from any of the plans, without limitation regarding pre-existing conditions. The employees make their choices during the open enrollment period. After that, they may not change plans until the next annual open enrollment season.

This program is administered by the **Office of Personnel Management (OPM).** The OPM requires that **each insurance company,** that offers a plan, meets certain minimum standards and provides a brochure. The brochure needs to describe the plan in plain English, using a standardized format for **easy comparison** of all the choices. It, also. must be downloadable in PDF format for online use.

When federal employees **retire at 65 years old** or older, they switch to Medicare, and their FEHB policy becomes their secondary insurance. If the employee continues to work after 65 years, the FEHB policy will remain the primary policy, and Medicare will be the secondary policy.

DEPARTMENT OF VETERANS AFFAIRS (VA), established in 1930, provides healthcare services for **veterans** who have been **discharged from active military service,** as long as it was **not a dishonorable discharge**. Certain benefits require that the veteran served during wartime. The veterans with a **service connected disability** are given **priority.** If the condition being treated by the VA, is military-related, no co-payment is required. However, any non military-related condition does require a co-payment.

ADMINISTRATION ON AGING (AoA) is a part of the **Department of Health and Human Services,** that provides funding to **assist home and community based programs,** to help older citizens and their caregivers. The AoA was created by the Older Americans Act (OAA) of 1965, which provides **grants to state and tribal organizations.** The **main objective,** of the OAA, is for older individuals to maintain their highest level of functional ability, so they can **remain in their own homes, for as long as possible.**

AoA provides multiple programs and services, through state administered **Area Agencies on Aging (AAA).** These programs and services include **nutritional services** (such as Meals on Wheels), **transportation services, adult day care, Alzheimer's Disease Support,** and **elder rights protection** (such as the **Ombudsmen** program). These services do not require the recipient to be living below the poverty level. However, the recipient may be asked, at no obligation, if they can make a donation for the services, to help keep the program viable.

The AAAs are comprised of a **network of local programs,** which provide outreach to older adults in the community. Each AAA is responsible for providing four key programs in their area. Those programs include health promotion, supportive services, nutritional programs, and caregiver support. **Health promotion** is accomplished through educational programs, such as fitness, nutrition, medication management, and disease management (such as diabetes and arthritis). **Supportive services** include educational materials, counseling, support groups, and respite services.

Family caregiver support programs include training, counseling, support groups, and respite services.

Besides home-delivered meals, congregate (community) meals are offered. An **important element** of the nutrition program is **socialization.** People, who need help getting their meals, are encouraged to **take advantage of the congregate meals,** because it provides other socializing activities, along with the meals. The **home-delivered meals** are mainly for homebound individuals, but even then, the volunteer who delivers the meals is trained to spend some time with the recipient. Sometimes, that volunteer is the only human contact the person has, on a regular basis.

Some agencies, also, receive funding from AoA, to provide **housekeeping services** for those older people, who because of illness or injury, were not able to do their own housekeeping. The service is limited, but sometimes is enough to help the individual avoid going into a nursing home or assisted living facility. This funding, also provides **some respite care,** so the caregiver might avoid experiencing burnout.

The **Ombudsman** program is administered by the individual states. Ombudsmen are trained to advocate for residents, located in their area, who are in skilled nursing facilities, assisted living facilities, and other elder care facilities. They visit adult care facilities, on a regular basis, to investigate and work to resolve complaints. They, also, provide training sessions for the facility staff to educate them about resident' rights. They function as a consultant for the facility staff, resident councils, and family councils.

The **AOA web site** provides search links, for elders and their families, to obtain information about available services in their communities. Access the **www.aoa.gov** web site, then click on the "Elders & Families" page. On that page, you will find several search links, including "**Find Local Programs**". That location will link you to the organization in your area and their web site.

REMINDER: Visit **www.aoa.gov** to see all the services available in your area. Another web site you can consult is the National Association of Area Agencies on Aging at **www.n4a.org**.

STATE DEPARTMENTS OF HEALTH SERVICES are responsible for the **regulation and licensing of various healthcare providers, within the state**. Facilities, regulated by this department, are nursing homes, assistive living facilities, behavioral health providers, child care, developmentally disabled group homes, juvenile group homes, emergency medical services, and medical facilities. Along with providing licenses for these services, it **sets performance standards** for these providers, which are posted on-line.

REMINDER: If you are utilizing any of these services, it is wise to become familiar with their **performance standards,** so you know what you can expect from them.

Besides licensing and setting standards, the Department of Health Services provides **onsite inspections and complaint investigations.** The Centers for Medicare and Medicaid Services also delegates to these state surveyors, the task of evaluating the various facilities for **Medicare and Medicaid certification**.

REMINDER: The **web sites** for the various state departments of health services. provide links for you to find health facilities, that are available in your area. They, also, provide information about **survey results** of the various facilities. This information could prove useful, when you need to select a healthcare provider.

STATE DEPARTMENTS OF ECONOMIC SECURITY (DES) are charged with the **safety and economic security of all the citizens of the state**. (Each state may have a variation on the title for this department.) Some of the health related services provided for Seniors, by this department, include **Adult Protective Services, Independent Living Programs, Long-Term Care, and Support for Caregivers.**

The general public is probably more familiar with Child Protective Services, than they are of **Adult Protective Services (APS).** This department **investigates** reports of neglect, abuse, or exploitation of **vulnerable adults,** and **reports any wrongdoing** to law enforcement. APS can also facilitate services to help protect vulnerable adults.

Common types of problems reported are "**self-neglect**" situations, where adults, due to physical and/or mental inability, are not able to meet their basic physical, medical, or financial needs. **Other examples** of situations, that may require a need to report, are when adults are **victims** of

neglect, financial exploitation, or physical, emotional, or sexual **abuse**.

Frequently, we think about reporting neglect or abuse, but forget about **financial exploitation**. Often, the vulnerable adult is being exploited by a family member. While providing home care, clients would comment to us, that they were missing money and couldn't afford to refill their medicine prescriptions. If this seemed to be a common occurrence for this client, we would report it, and let the APS investigator decide if this was a true situation of exploitation.

My cousin spent her career as an accountant. She kept close watch over where her money went. She did discover that one of the aides, at the assisted living facility, took a couple of checks from the bottom of her checkbook, and tried to forge them. Fortunately, her bank observed that the signatures, on the checks, did not match her signature on file.

REMINDER: If you know of a situation that may indicate a possibility of abuse, neglect, or exploitation, it **should be reported**. Your name will be kept **confidential.** The agency is **responsible to do their own investigation.** Therefore, any actions taken will not be, solely, based on your input.

Independent living programs, include services that help individuals remain in their homes, rather than needing to move into a nursing care facility. These **services can include** case management, home care, housekeeping services, adult day care, respite care, transportation, community meals, and home-delivered meals. Frequently, just one or two of these services, could make the difference between living at home or moving to a care facility. These services are **provided** by the state department, **in conjunction with** the Agency on Aging (AOA). **Eligibility** for these services **is not** based upon income, but is **based upon disability**.

There are many disabled adults, who are able to continue living in their homes, thanks to **care giving services** provided by family members or friends. The stress of caring for a loved one can be overwhelming. The states try to **help the in-home caregivers** by providing information, help to gain access to supportive care (such as nursing aide services or nursing visits), support groups, caregiver training, respite care, and supplemental services, such as housekeeping.

Another program, administered by a state DES, is the **State Health Insurance Assistance Programs (SHIP).** These programs are funded by the Centers for Medicare and Medicaid Services and the Administration on Aging. The program provides **counselors,** to help Medicare beneficiaries and their families make informed decisions about Medicare enrollment and supplemental insurance coverage. These counselors are trained in Medicare and Medicaid law and regulations, and health insurance products. They are **not connected to insurance companies or licensed to sell insurance**. This program will play a role in the implementation of the Affordable Care Act of 2010, which will be discussed in more detail latter in this book.

CHAPTER III

PRIVATE MEDICAL INSURANCE

Private insurances, originally, were intended to be used for catastrophic medical events. Now most people have come to depend on it (even expect it) for routine medical care. When big businesses started to pay for employee's healthcare, it was viewed as a special benefit; now many employees consider it an entitlement.

Initially, employees were expected to pay for part of their medical care, **but now** some of the programs do not require a co-payment, or the payment is minimal. Many healthcare providers feel, when individuals pay nothing or little for their healthcare, they are less likely to take responsibility for their health.

Insurances can be **categorized** under various classifications, such as **PPO** (preferred provider organization), **HMO** (health maintenance organization), **Managed Care**, **Fee for Service,** or **Third Party Payer**. Many of these types of insurance were developed in an effort to control health care costs.

MANAGED CARE:

This is a term used to described various programs, that have been designed to **control healthcare costs.** Like many other programs, "it sounded good on paper", but it also created some unanticipated problems. One problem was that insurance companies started to **determine what was acceptable healthcare treatment,** instead of allowing the physician and patient to make these decisions. This situation has improved, as patients and healthcare professionals, have learned to communicate with the insurance companies.

Some of the **mechanisms, used** to reduce healthcare costs, are **controls** on hospital admissions and lengths of stay, and **emphasis** on preventive care. Additionally, **incentives** to use outpatient services and other less costly forms of care are employed. The desire to improve the management of healthcare costs took on many different forms, such as HMOs and PPOs.

REMINDER: No matter what type of insurance program you buy into, be sure to read over the policy carefully, so you understand the rules. Keep a copy of the policy handy, so you can refer to it when you have questions about your healthcare.

Health Maintenance Organizations (HMO):

This first form of managed care was developed in the 1970s. In addition to providing financial support of healthcare, HMOs deliver healthcare services.

The **original idea** was, for the payment of **a monthly fee,** the HMO would work to **keep the client healthy,** through routine medical visits, education, and preventive care. If the patient **required further treatment or hospitalization,** the HMO would **provide it without further cost** to the patient. In the beginning, most HMOs provided the direct medical care. A **disadvantage** was that HMOs were not available in all communities. Another disadvantage, for the HMO, was if there were more than the anticipated number of patients requiring major medical care. As the HMO's patient population grew older, the medical care became more expensive. Over the years, **HMOs have modified their practices** to, both, meet the needs of their patients and to remain financially solvent.

Today, there are about **three general types of HMOs**. One type is the **staff model,** which employs the medical staff to see HMO patients only, in an HMO facility. This type usually runs their own hospitals.

The second type of HMO is the **group model**. This HMO contracts with a group of physicians, with a variety of specialties, who are employed by the group. These physicians see other patients, beside the HMO patients. A variance to this model is a captive group model, which only cares for HMO patients.

Another variance of the group model is the **Independent Practice Association (IPA)**. With this type of association, private practice physicians may contract with an IPA, and still maintain their independent practice.

The third type of HMO is a **network model.** With this model, the HMO contracts with any combination of groups. Since the 1990s, most HMOs have been operating under the network model, which has made HMOs more available to most communities.

Basically, HMOs **contract with physicians and other healthcare professionals,** to care for their clients. These professionals are required to **follow the HMO's guidelines and restrictions.** The HMO members are required to select **a primary care physician (PCP),** who will act as a "**gatekeeper**". The PCP provides the **basic medical care** and makes **referrals to specialists,** when needed. The HMO, usually, will not cover any specialty care that was not referred by the PCP.

HMOs provide healthcare at lower cost for the patient, with a **focus on wellness and preventive care.** Disadvantages of the HMO system are **limitations** on **choice** of a **primary physician** and limited **specialized care**.

Preferred Provider Organization (PPO):
Another type of managed care, the PPO, is a **group of physicians** and/or other healthcare providers that **contract with a health insurance agency,** to provide healthcare at a reduced rate. The patient is responsible for **paying the annual deductible and co-payments,** whereas, the insurance company will pay for the rest of the care to the provider. The patient is allowed to utilize an out-of-network provider, but must pay a higher amount, pay the provider directly, and then obtain reimbursement from the insurance company.

PPOs provide **freer choice** of a healthcare provider, and out-of-pocket expenses are limited. There is less financial coverage for care, if out-of-network providers are utilized, with more expense and paperwork for the services. Some people feel the extra work and expense is worth it, in exchange for the freedom of choosing their own healthcare provider.

POINT OF SERVICE (POS):

POS Combines the characteristics of HMOs and PPOs. There are no deductible payments, but there could be limited co-payments. The patient is required to see a **primary care physician**, who makes **referrals within the POS** network. The individual can choose a healthcare provider outside the network, but will be charged a deductible and, possibly, increased co-payments.

An POS allows the **greatest freedom** among the three types of managed care, when choosing a provider. The out-of-pocket costs are limited, especially if the patient remains within the network. There does tend to be tighter controls for specialized care.

SPECIALTY HEALTHCARE INSURANCES:

These insurances take on **many forms,** including ones for cancer treatment and long-term care insurance. One type I recommend to my family and friends, especially as they get older, is **long-term care insurance.** Many people assume that Medicare and their secondary insurance will cover all their needs. That may be true, if you or your spouse do not ever need to utilize extended care, in a nursing home or at home.

Medicare and regular health insurance policies do not pay for custodial type care. **Custodial care** is when the patient requires assistance with their activities of daily living, such as bathing, eating, or keeping safe, but does not require some type of skilled care from a nurse or therapist. These non-skilled expenses have led to bankruptcy for many people.

As discussed earlier, there is always **Medicaid** which **does pay for custodial care**, to fall back on. However, most of us prefer not to go in that direction, if it can be avoided. Also, there are some of us that would not qualify for Medicaid. Most **long-term insurances** will help cover home care, assisted living care homes, or skilled nursing facilities.

I was sorry my cousin, Em, did not get long-term insurance, but once she was admitted to a Skilled Nursing Facility, it was too late. She could have purchased the insurance any time before her admission to the care facility. Even though it would have been expensive, it would have helped her with her bills, and she probably could have avoided running out of money. The longer you wait, the higher the premiums.

Along with providing help with medical bills, frequently, insurance companies are able to negotiate a better room and board rate. If Em could have paid the rate that Medicaid negotiated for their clients, she would not have run out of money. (It would have been close to $2000 cheaper per month.) **Private pay patients** are at a **disadvantage,** when trying to negotiate a reasonable room and care rate.

REMINDER: Seriously consider purchasing long-term care insurance. The sooner you do it, the better the premium rate you will get.

The 2010 HEALTHCARE BILL (PATIENT PROTECTION AND AFFORDABLE CARE ACT):

Has a few portions that are being implemented, within the first year of enactment, but the major parts of the bill will not be implemented until **2014.**

One area, of implementation, is the elimination of **preexisting disease restriction.** Uninsured individuals, with preexisting conditions, may be able to qualify for new coverage. The Department of Health and Human Services has established a temporary Preexisting Condition Insurance Plan (PCIP) for those uninsured Americans, who have been unable to obtain coverage, due to a preexisting health condition.

Beginning September 23, 2010, preexisting condition exclusions were no longer allowed for new insurance policies for children under the age of 19 years. The **goal is to eventually** eliminate preexisting condition exclusions **for all age groups**. The PCIP is intended to cover the eligible uninsured adults, until January 1, 2014, when, hopefully, there will be more non-governmental insurance programs available for these individuals.

Beginning **September 23, 2010,** new insurance policies will be prohibited from having "**lifetime dollar limits**". Annual dollar limits will gradually be phased out, between September 2010 and 2014.

Another aspect of the 2010 plan, to go into early effect, is the continued **coverage of young adults, under the age of 26 years,** on their parents' insurance plans. Beginning **September 23, 2010**, parents can cover their adult children on their policies, if that policy allows dependent coverage. An exception, would be, if young adults can obtain their own health insurance through their job.

When first created, **Medicare Part D** (the Drug benefit) contained a **coverage gap**, referred to as the **"donut hole".** The 2010 Healthcare Bill hopes to, **eventually, close that gap**. Beginning in June 2010, individuals who have Part D coverage, will receive a $250 rebate when they reach the coverage gap. The plan is, that **beginning in 2011**, individuals who reach the "donut hole", will get a 50% discount on certain designated brand-name medications.

Another objective, of the Affordable Care Act, is to **foster wellness and preventive care practices,** by eliminating deductibles and co-payments for preventive services. Some of these services, include **screening** for cardiac disease, diabetes, and cancer, **counseling** for smoking cessation and addictive behavior, and assistance for weight loss. Another aspect of this program would be providing **immunizations** for childhood diseases, flu, and pneumonia. .

The Bill calls for the establishment of **health insurance exchanges, by 2014,** and a more standardized and uniform appeals process for any new insurance plans. This will include an **internet portal** to provide easy access for information about affordable coverage, in an easy-to-read, uniform format, that will **foster comparison** of the various insurance policies.

REMINDER: For more details about the 2010 Healthcare Bill, go to **www.healthcare.gov.**

QUESTIONS to consider when you are selecting a new Medical Insurance Provider.

What Physicians will I be able to see?

Do I need a primary care physician?

Is there a good selection of primary care providers from which to choose?

What medical services will be covered?

What out-of-pocket expenses will there be?

Will emergency care be covered?

Am I required to stay within a certain network?

Are the network services readily available?

What are the reputations of the in-network providers?

Do I need a referral to see a specialist?

How long do you have to wait for an   appointment?

How much time does your PCP spend with you when you have an appointment?

Am I allowed an opportunity to interview the provider before making a decision?

Does your provider remember you and your medical conditions each time you see him/her?

Do you see the same provider whenever you have a medical appointment?

How long do you have to wait to see the physician when you have an appointment?

If you have a long wait (more than 20-30 minutes), does anyone show any concern or give an explanation?

CHAPTER IV

HEALTHCARE STATEMENTS/ BILLS INTERPRETATION

Always read over your medical statements carefully, even if you do not have to make any payments. You want to be sure the proper charges are being made for the **appropriate procedures.** Most healthcare workers are honest, but there are some people who try to make fraudulent charges. Also, there are others who might make an honest mistake.

Medical charges are submitted, when billing Medicare or insurance companies, by using a variety of **codes,** depending upon the medical situation. Considering the number and variety of codes that are used, it is not difficult to make an error. **You are the one most** likely to notice a discrepancy in the billing.

Three common codes used for billing are CPT (Current Procedural Terminology), ICD (International Classification of Diseases), and DRG (Diagnosis Related Groups). Medical codes are used to describe treatments and diseases, and help categorize them.

The **CPT codes** were developed, by the American Medical Association, to describe all of the healthcare services. **ICD codes** are maintained by the CDC (Centers for Disease Control) and the World Health Association. These codes, which change frequently, describe **medical diseases and variations,** such as one code for diabetes and another for diabetes with a wound. There are hundreds of ICD codes and variations.

The **DRGs** were developed by Medicare to classify **groups of hospitalized patients.** These, approximately 500 groups, are used to determine reimbursement for hospitalization. It is assumed that all patients, within a particular group (heart attack), would require the same medical services. The DRGs are revised from time to time, but not as frequently as the ICD codes.

The code revisions do contribute to confusion with billings. Healthcare billing has become so complicated that there is a **special healthcare degree** for individuals, who specialize in medical coding.

If you do find a discrepancy in your bill, phone your medical provider first. They are entitled to know if you have a question, that might be easy to resolve. Some discrepancies can be caused by entering a wrong number, and could be easy to correct. If not satisfied, then you can make further contacts. You want to be fair, but you are, also, entitled to have your questions answered.

Many times people become upset about charges, when reading their medical bills. For example, when someone has been hospitalized, they get upset when they look at their itemized bills, and question the expense of the room or certain supplies.

Room rates look expensive because they **include** the cost of the **nursing staff and other personnel** who care for you, while you are a patient. As a nurse, I dislike the idea that a hospital bill never reflects the nursing care, so crucial for the safe recovery of hospitalized patients.

The **cost of supplies** includes, not only the particular supply, such as a dressing, but also, the **nurse who changed** that dressing. In addition, the dressing is listed by the brand name, i.e. Band Aid. When people see that name, they imagine the small band aid, that is used on a small cut at home, and wonder why it is so expensive. **Medication** prices reflect the **pharmacist,** who sets up the doses, and the **nurse,** who administers the medication.

There are times when a mistake is made on a patient's bill, so it is good to **ask for an itemized bill,** and look it over to be sure it is accurate. If there is a question, the facility's billing department should be your first call.

Current practices of healthcare reimbursement have evolved in the past decades, in an effort to contain costs. The **Centers for Medicare and Medicaid,** of the Federal Government, has set up regulations defining **conditions of participation,** that must be met to receive reimbursement for medical services.

Medical insurance companies have adopted some of these same regulations, to varying degrees. Many insurance and Medicaid organizations require medical professionals to **obtain either verbal or written approval** for medical procedures, before the services can be provided. Some of these measures have helped control medical costs, however, some of these practices have increased the time spent on non-medical tasks and less on patient care.

CHAPTER V

HEALTHCARE CARE PROVIDERS

Primary Care Providers (PCP)

Primary care providers are medical professionals who are licensed, by a given state, to **provide independent medical care**. Each state may have some variance on which professionals are allowed to practice as a PCP.

To add to the confusion, some of **these titles** may have **more than one meaning.** For example: a given state may consider **all physicians** to be primary care physicians. Another state or insurance provider would consider **only the general practitioner or internist** to be the primary care provider. That would mean, if you bypassed one of the designated providers, and went directly to a specialist, the **services might not be covered** by your insurance or one of the federal programs.

This shows the **importance of always asking questions,** and not making assumptions. Of course, you might think: "But what if I don't know what questions to ask?" This is one reason why I decided this book needed to be written. The book may not give you all of the answers, but it will provide **resources, to help you find answers**.

Most specialists will **try to keep you informed** about the rules, but sometimes, they may not realize you bypassed the primary care provider. Other times, they may think you were already informed of the rules, or they may use some medical jargon that you did not understand. I have noticed many times that when someone does not understand something, they **hate to appear "dumb",** so they smile and nod, as if they understand what is being said.

REMINDER: Do not be afraid to **ask questions**. Always write down a **list of questions** you want to ask the doctor, and **then use** your list. **Don't feel guilty,** that you may be "holding up" the doctor with your questions; it is **their responsibility** to answer them.

In addition to licensed **Medical Doctors (MD),** primary care physicians include **Osteopathic Physicians (DO).** Many states, also, license **Nurse Practitioners (NP)** as primary care providers.

Primary care practitioners function as **gatekeepers,** who refer their patients to the appropriate specialists, when needed, and navigate those patients through the healthcare system. They **collaborate and coordinate** their patients' healthcare with specialists and other healthcare providers.

The PCPs' **scope of practice** includes **diagnosis and treatment of common medical conditions**. They provide generalized healthcare, which includes **health maintenance and preventive healthcare** measures, such as diet instruction, and vaccinations for flu and pneumonia.

REMINDER: Be sure to **keep your PCP informed** about any **new medications** and **treatments** you are receiving, including over the counter medications. Some people, who go to more than one healthcare provider, could be taking two or more medications that have similar actions. Essentially, they could be in danger of receiving an **overdose** of the medication.

Our country has a **limited number of PCPs,** for various reasons. One reason is the reimbursement rate for the general practitioner tends to be less, than for a specialist. Also, there are some areas of the country, such as **rural areas,** that experience a critical shortage of PCPs.

This shortage is expected to worsen. Medical school students indicate their preference to pursue a medical specialty, rather than general practitioner or family medicine. Also, most of them indicate they plan to practice in a metropolitan area, rather than a rural area.

Hence, the **nurse practitioner** has filled a much needed service, as a PCP. The nurse practitioner's **scope of practice varies, according to the** regulations within the state in which the NP is practicing. Some states require the NP to work in collaboration with a physician, whereas in other states, the NP practices independently.

REMEMBER: It is wise to **become established with a PCP,** even if you feel healthy. **Keep follow-up visits** with your PCP, especially if you have a chronic condition, such as diabetes or heart disease. It is important, to have an **annual physical,** even if you are healthy. If you do not keep your annual visit, you may be required to find another PCP. Also, your annual physical **could reveal** a developing condition, of which you were not aware.

TYPES of PRIMARY CARE PRACTITIONERS

The **Physician** is either a graduate of a **school of Medicine (MD)** or a school of **Osteopathy (DO)**. In the United States, the physician completes an approved residency program and successfully completes medical boards. Physicians, who have attended medical school in a foreign country, must complete the medical boards and participate in a residency program (3-7 years) at an approved institution in the United States.

Frequently, the MD is **board certified in a specialty area**. These certification boards do include a board for the family physician and for the general practitioner. Physicians use the **medical model** in their practice. In other words, their focus is on the physical and biological aspects of a patient's disease or medical condition.

The **Nurse Practitioner** is a registered nurse, who has completed **advanced nursing education.** The requirements for the NP varies from state to state. Most states require a **minimum of a master's degree in nursing,** with a **specialty as a nurse practitioner**. Many NPs have, also, completed a Ph.D or Doctorate in nursing.

Frequently, nurse practitioners specialize in a particular area of health care. Examples of these areas are pediatrics, maternity, family health, or elder care. Some of these areas **require additional experience and certification.**

The NP is prepared to **diagnose and treat common medical conditions**. They **collaborate** with physicians and other healthcare professionals, to treat the patient. They have an **expertise in patient and family education and counseling.**

States vary in their authorization for NPs to **independently prescribe medications.** Most states do authorize them to prescribe medications and interpret lab value results, as well. Some require that their orders be cosigned by a physician.

NPs provide **health maintenance and preventive health** care. Most patients are very happy with their services, especially since the NP takes time to listen to them, and explain their condition and treatment in detail.

Nurse Practitioners tend to **utilize the nursing model** in their practice. The nursing model uses a **holistic approach**. In other words, they not only consider the physical manifestations of the patient's condition, but also emotional and social aspects.

GENERALISTS and SPECIALISTS

General Practitioners (GP) are physicians who, after completion of their internship/residency, choose to remain in **general (family) practice.** As stated previously, there are insufficient numbers of GPs to service the needs, especially, with our growing senior population, and, most especially, in rural and low income areas.

Internists provide medical treatment for conditions that involve the **internal systems of the body**. Internists, frequently, are primary care physicians.

Pediatricians specialize in the medical care of children, from **birth to young adulthood.**

Obstetricians/ Gynecologists specialize in **women's health.** An obstetrician's care is focused on **childbirth,** whereas, gynecologists provide general medical care for **female conditions**, other than childbirth. Some of these physicians practice in both areas.

Psychiatrists are physicians who assess and treat **mental illness, and promote mental health.**

Surgeons specialize in the **treatment of injuries, disease, and deformities, through surgery.** Some surgeons perform general surgery, while others specialize in orthopedics (musculoskeletal), neurological (brain & nervous system), and cardiovascular (heart & vessels), to name a few.

Some of the **many medical specialties** are cardiology (heart), dermatology (skin), gastroenterology (stomach & intestines), ophthalmology (eye), oncology (cancer), pathology (laboratory analysis & medical examination), and radiology (x-ray/imaging).

These are just a few types of specialties available to physicians. No wonder we get confused about which doctor we should see, when we are ill. This is one reason why we need to have a primary care professional.

A relatively new specialty is the **Hospitalist**. A hospitalist is a physician whose focus is the care of the **hospitalized patient**. The term was first identified in 1996.

Approximately, half of the country's community hospitals utilize this specialty. Factors that have promoted the use of this specialist include the multiple medical problems of hospital patients and the need to **coordinate care** of the patient **between all the specialists,** who may be writing orders for the individual. Primary care physicians have found value in turning their patient's care over to a **hospitalist,** who can be **readily available** to the patient and, also. **free up the primary physician** to see more patients in the office.

Some hospitalists specialize in providing care in a **specific area** of the hospital, such as the intensive care unit. They provide 24/7 care to patients in that area. Because the hospitalist is such a new specialty, many patients are not aware of their existence, and are **taken by surprise** when they are hospitalized under the care of someone other than their primary care physician. Patients are **entitled to be informed** by their primary physician, if their care is to be turned over to a hospitalist when they are admitted to the hospital. Hospitalists **initiate orders** for the patient, when they are being discharged, but the primary care physician needs to provide any follow-up orders and care.

REMINDER: Make sure you or a family member **contacts your primary care physician,** when you are discharged from the hospital, to ensure there is no delay in needed follow-up care. If you **do not have a primary care provider**, you are **responsible** to find one after discharge.

Board Certification is required by most specialty areas. The **requirements** for achieving board certification status varies, depending on the specialty. After completion of a residency program in the specialty, the physician is required to complete some additional requirements, that may include **assessment of clinical performance** and a **written certification examination**. Some specialty boards require the candidate to have a period of full-time practice, of at least 2 years, before taking the examination. The examination process may also include an oral exam. Some of the boards require **periodic recertification**, usually every 7 to 10 years. Recertification requirements usually include proof of continuing education, review of credentials, and reexamination.

OTHER HEALTHCARE PROVIDERS

There are two types of **Nurses:** Licensed (LPN or LVN) and Registered (RN). The **title "Nurse"** is a legal title. In most states, this term is **to be used only** in conjunction with an RN or LPN. There are some unlicensed individuals who call themselves a nurse and should not be using that title. An example is medical assistants, who work in physicians' offices. It is wise to **clarify,** that they are actually a nurse and, if so, which type

The **Licensed Nurse** may be titled either **Licensed Practical (LPN)** or **Licensed Vocational (LVN)** nurse, depending on the state in which they practice. The PN/VN has completed at least a **1-year nursing program,** and passed the **State Board Examination for the LPN/LVN.** The board examination for LN is the same nationwide test, which provides consistency in licensure, from state to state. Practical nurses are **licensed in the state,** in which they practice. They must always practice **under the supervision** of a registered nurse or a physician. They are prepared to provide **basic bedside care**, monitor and record patient vital signs, perform **procedures**, administer oral and injectable **medications,** and help **teach basic routine health care**. Licensed nurses work in all types of healthcare settings. Experienced LPNs supervise aides in a nursing home setting. Because of constantly changing healthcare information, they are expected to participate in continuing education, and update their nursing skills.

The **Registered Nurse (RN)** is educated in either an **associate degree program ADN (2-year), bachelor of science degree program BSN (4-year), or diploma program (3-year).** Today, most RNs graduate from either an ADN or BSN program. Many RNs continue their education, to move from ADN to BSN and even on to a **master degree in nursing (MSN).** On-line nursing programs, have facilitated the ability of nurses to further their education, while still working. There are, also, **doctoral and Ph.D** programs available in nursing.

Upon graduation from an approved nursing program, the graduate takes the **NCLEX-RN** test for licensure, which is accepted by all US states. The RN is prepared to **practice independently,** in **multiple work settings.** Besides hospitals, RNs practice in clinics, doctors' offices, home care, skilled nursing facilities, elementary and secondary schools, and hospice care. Nurses, with advanced degrees, may go into nursing education, hospital or nursing home management, or advanced clinical practice. RNs are **licensed** by the **individual state,** where they practice.

When caring for patients, RNs establish a **holistic plan of care,** by assessing patient's physical and psychosocial data, planning and implementing the care, observing for and preventing complications, and evaluating the results. Besides providing **nursing care**, they **advocate** for their patients and **teach** them and their families about their conditions, medications, nutrition, treatments, and general health. They administer oral, injectable, and intravenous **medications**. They insert and monitor intravenous injections, nasogastric tubes, and urinary catheters. They perform a variety of **highly technical treatments,** including wound care.

There are many **Therapists** involved in providing healthcare. This book will focus on the therapists who are licensed, and prepared to practice independently. The three major groups are Physical, Occupational, and Speech-Language Therapists. This section will give an overview of each group's focus, and licensing requirements. Later chapters will discuss more specifics of their practice, in relation to the various health care venues, and medical conditions.

Physical Therapists (PT) are prepared to develop,. maintain, and/or restore maximum ability for **movement and function,** when disability is related to aging, injury, disease, or environment. The PT **develops a management plan,** that may include exercise, manual therapy, education, and other interventions. The PT bases the management plan on the individual's history and physical exam.

PTs **function independently in many venues,** including hospitals, nursing homes, home care, and outpatient clinics. They work with **all age groups,** and treat clients with **various medical conditions** and **disabilities**, including cardiac (heart), neurological (brain, spinal cord, nerves), orthopedic (bones), muscular, and skin conditions.

The PT's practice is **regulated** by the **individual states,** in which they practice. Today, a new PT must be a graduate from an **accredited physical therapy program,** with either a **master's or doctoral degree** in PT. Gaining admission into a PT program is highly competitive. These programs include academic and clinical components. A PT graduate must pass the **National PT examination,** to become licensed. Many states require a certain number of **continuing education** hours to maintain licensure.

Occupational Therapists (OT) promote health of individuals and groups, through occupation. **Occupation** does not just mean how one **earns a living,** but also includes **leisure** activities, **self care**, **domestic,** and **community** activities.

The occupational therapist is a professional, who **functions independently,** in many areas of the community. Some of these areas include schools, prisons, rehabilitation facilities, mental health, skilled nursing facilities, and home health agencies. OTs work with clients who experience **mental, physical, developmental,** and/or **emotional disabilities**. The OTs' focus is to assist their clients **achieve independence** in all areas of their lives.

To practice in the US, an OT must earn a **masters degree** or greater from an occupational therapy program. The OT must be **licensed.** The OT license requires that the individual has graduated from an **accredited OT program** and passed the **National Certification Examination of Occupational Therapy.**

Speech-Language Pathologists (SLP) work with clients, who are dealing with issues concerning **speech, language, and/or communication disorders**. These disorders include **cognitive and swallowing** impairments.

They **function independently** in a **wide range of settings,** including schools, hospitals, clinics, skilled nursing facilities, and home health agencies. Some of the **medical disorders,** that require a SLP, include hearing loss, stroke (CVA), cerebral palsy, brain injury, and cancer.

Certification of Clinical Competence, in Speech-Language Pathology, requires a **Masters Degree in Speech Pathology, 375 hours of supervised clinical** experience, passage of the **National Speech-Language Pathology examination,** and at least **9 months of post graduate experience**. Also, there is a mandatory **3-year license renewal** required with demonstration of continued competence.

Pharmacists' main responsibilities relate to the **dispensing of prescription medications**. They, also, **provide information** to the consumer about drug actions, administration, side effects, precautions, adverse reactions, interactions, and incompatibilities.

It helps if consumers have all their prescriptions filled at the same pharmacy, because the pharmacist can then **monitor for adverse interactions** between all of the consumer's medications. Pharmacists **advise physicians and other**

health care professionals about drug dosages, interactions, and side effects. They are prepared to **answer questions** about diabetes, asthma, hypertension, and other chronic conditions that are controlled by drug therapy.

A pharmacist, in the US, must complete a **4 year graduate program in pharmacy.** Candidates must have **at least two years of undergraduate education,** which includes math and sciences. However, most pharmacy candidates have a bachelor's degree, before entering their pharmacy program. Upon graduation, pharmacists must pass the **North American Pharmacist Licensure Exam** and a **pharmacy law exam**. Some pharmacists are board certified in a **specialty area,** such as nuclear medicine, nutritional, oncological (cancer therapy), psychiatric, and geriatric pharmacy.

REMINDER: Be sure to **read the literature** that accompanies your medications, and **pay attention to any precautions** printed on the label of your medication container.

Social Workers (BSW/MSW) can be found practicing in a **variety of settings,** such as schools, correctional areas, mental health, hospitals, medical clinics, home care, skilled nursing, assisted living, community centers, or independent practice. Social workers function as **case managers, community organizers, sociology teachers, and counselors.** They make **referrals,** teach **coping skills,** help with **problem solving**, **advocate** for clients, **seek out resources** for the client, and guide them in the use of these resources.

Social work education programs vary from a **bachelor's to a Ph.D degree**. In most states, one must have a minimum of a **master's degree** to function **independently**. Often, they must have a **license or be registered** as a social worker.

Physician Assistant (PA) is a relatively new medical profession. The first PA program was established in 1965, in response to physician shortages and their uneven availability in certain communities. PAs are **licensed to practice medicine, under the supervision** of a physician.

Their **scope of practice varies,** according to the physician's specialty. PAs are prepared to perform physical exams, diagnose illnesses, interpret lab tests, treat illnesses, assist in surgeries, and write prescriptions. Their scope of practice varies from state to state. Some states require that their orders be co-signed by their supervising physician, while other states do not require a co-signature.

They do not practice on the physician's license, but have **their own licenses.** Most PA educational programs require students to already have **health experience** and **some college** education. Many candidates have a bachelor's degree in another area. The **PA educational programs** vary in length, from certificate programs to master's degree programs. **Certification** requires graduation from an **accredited PA program** and passage of the **National Certification examination**. The PA is required to earn 100 hours in **continuing education, re-register** their certificates **every 2 years,** and **recertify every 6 years** by successfully completing a National Recertification exam.

Therapy Assistants & Aides work under the **supervision of a Licensed Therapist.** There are therapy assistants and aides for physical, occupational, and speech-language therapy.

After the therapist develops a plan of care for the client, the **Therapy Assistant** will **aide** with the **implementation** of that plan by providing exercises, treatments, documentation, and education. They also contribute information, to the therapist, to help in the development of the plan of care.

Although they work under the supervision of the therapist, the therapist does not need to provide direct supervision. In other words, the therapist does not need to be in the immediate area, where the assistant is functioning. However, the therapist is responsible to know that the assistant is providing **safe and appropriate care,** and is following the client's **plan of care**.

Therapy assistants have a minimum of an **associate degree (2-year) in the discipline** of which they are working (physical, occupational, or speech-language therapy). Most states regulate therapy assistants through **licensing, certification, or registration.** Some states, also, require proof of continuing education to maintain their status.

Therapy Aides usually receive "**on-the-job**" **training,** and must work under **direct supervision** of the therapist. Their job responsibilities consist, mainly, of **clerical** work, and readying the **treatment area and equipment** for the therapy sessions. Therapy aides are not qualified to participate in providing the actual therapy. However, they may assist in the **transport of the client** to and from the treatment area. Aides are not individually regulated by the state, however, each state does regulate the operation of healthcare facilities which utilize the therapy aide.

Certified Nursing Assistants (CNA) should always work under the **supervision of a nurse**, either RN or LPN, depending on the work setting. CNAs can be found functioning in **most healthcare settings,** such as hospitals, skilled nursing facilities, assisted living, hospice, and home care.

Basically, CNAs **assist patients** carry out their **activities of daily living,** such as bathing, dressing, eating, elimination, and mobility. They are also qualified to take **vital signs**, such as blood pressure, pulse, and temperatures.

Out of concern for safe elder care, the Federal Government set some minimal requirements for the education of the CNA. The CNA program must be **at least 75 hours** in length, and include **classroom** instruction. **Laboratory** practice and supervised **clinical** experience are included in the course. They are **certified** within the state they practice, after passing written and practical examinations.

CNAs are, also, required to have at least **12 hours of continuing education** per year. Some states allow non-certified aides to practice in certain healthcare venues. Most states require that only CNAs (not uncertified aides) can provide care in skilled nursing facilities and general hospitals/ medical centers.

CHAPTER VI

STAYING HEALTHY I

Many of us are living longer lives than, even our parents did, thanks to better healthcare, increased health awareness, and improved access to nutritional food. But there are some dangers lurking in the future, if we are not careful. As we get older, we need to work harder to maintain our health.

There are many resources available to help us sustain our health, but we are "our main resource". In other words, we **must take responsibility** for our health. Usually, those who get **regular exercise**, eat a **balanced diet**, **avoid addictive behavior,** and maintain **regular healthcare visits,** tend to retain better physical, emotional, and mental health.

We know we can remain healthier through **regular exercise** and a **balanced diet.** We cannot depend on, just taking a pill, to remain healthy.

As everyone should be well aware, obesity is a major problem in all age groups. **Obesity,** not only, reflects an individual's lifestyle, but it is, also, an indication of susceptibility for some underlying medical conditions, such as diabetes, joint disease, and cardiac disease.

NUTRITION

Nutrition plays a major role in staying healthy. Each individual has special issues in relation to their nutrition.

Weight control is, probably, the most common issue for senior citizens. Some seniors have the problem of being overweight, while others have the opposite problem, of being underweight. Overcoming the underweight problem can be just as difficult, as overcoming too much weight. If you have a nutritional problem, it helps to begin by keeping a **food diary** of your eating habits.

There is so much conflicting information about nutrition today, it is not surprising that one gets confused about what constitutes a "good" or balanced diet. All of the **basic nutrients** (water, protein, fats, carbohydrates/starches, minerals, & vitamins) **are important** to include in the daily diet. Whether you need to gain, lose, or maintain weight, will dictate whether you need to increase or decrease particular nutrients, such as carbohydrates.

There are many **resources** you can use to help manage your diet, including those found online. If you have special dietary needs, especially related to a medical condition, the best resource would be a **dietitian or nutritionist.** Your doctor or local healthcare facility can help direct you toward that resource.

Senior citizens experience **changes with aging** that can affect their dietary needs. Physical changes include reduced taste, digestive disturbances, and reduced mobility.

Over the years, the US population has become more faithful in practicing good dental health care, which has resulted in less need for dentures. Those who do need **dentures,** may experience more difficulty while **chewing** their food, especially if the dentures fit poorly. People with dentures have difficulty chewing tough meats, fresh fruits, and vegetables. They also tend to experience **reduced taste** because of the presence of dentures.

Some senior citizens, even those who don't need dentures, experience **changes in taste of salt and sugar.** The reduction in the sense of taste for salt may prompt the individual to use excess amounts of it. Rather than increasing the amount of salt, which can be dangerous, the use of other spices, such as cinnamon, may be helpful.

Food tolerances may also change for seniors. Some people find they experience problems with diarrhea, constipation, or indigestion with certain foods. Avoidance of spicy foods may be helpful. Stool softeners and extra fluids may help with constipation.

Increased **dry mouth,** caused by aging and/or certain oral medications, can also be a problem. Drinking water and using mouthwash can help. Use of artificial saliva agents may, also, be useful in severe cases.

Some elders experience **reduced mobility,** due to joint changes, weakness, or complications of a physical disorder. This can affect one's nutrition by the mere fact that it is **difficult obtaining and/or preparing food.** Sometimes it is easier to **eat a donut,** than prepare a salad. The problem can be compounded if the individual is on a **fixed income.** It is cheaper to fill up on the **less expensive starche**s, such as bread, rice, or potatoes, rather than vegetables and meat.

Constipation is a common complaint among senior citizens. This can be due to a variety of factors. **Three factors** that help maintain normal bowel function are **physical activity, fluids, and adequate fiber** in the diet. If something interferes with maintaining one of these factors, it helps to increase the other two. So if you develop a condition that interferes with your mobility, it will help if you increase your fluid and fiber intake in your diet. **Water** is the best fluid you can drink. Be aware that some drinks, such as coffee, can actually be a dehydrator. Good **sources of fiber** include vegetables, whole grain breads, and cereals. **Stool softeners and/or laxatives** may help prevent constipation. Be careful not to overuse laxatives, as they can become habit forming.

REMINDER: If you have a deficiency in one of the three factors that promote bowel function (exercise, fluids, fiber), **increase your use** of the other two factors to compensate.

Major Foods/ Nutrients, that all age groups need to include in their diets, consist of carbohydrates, fruits, protein, vegetables, fats, fiber, minerals, and water. The importance of the various nutrients change as one ages, and the lack of them could lead to a chronic medical condition.

Carbohydrates:

- **Include** sugars, starches, and fiber.
- Granulated sugars and fruit juices are included in the **sugar** category.
- Examples of **starches** are breads, potatoes, noodles, and rice.
- **Fiber** sources include whole grains, vegetables, and fruits, such as prunes and figs.
- Carbohydrates **provide energy** to the body, and help **regulate blood sugar**.
- It is **recommended** that individuals consume per day:
  - 4-5 servings of grains/starches,
  - 2-3 servings of vegetables (especially the green leafy type),
  - 2-4 servings of fruits.
- **Examples of serving sizes are:**
  - **Grains/starches:** 1 slice of bread, 1 cup dry cereal, 1/2 cup rice or pasta,
  - **Vegetables**: 1/2 cup juice or cut vegetables, 1 cup leafy vegetables,

Proteins:

- **Include** meats, fish, eggs, beans, nuts, soy products, and dairy products.
- Protein is used in the body as building blocks **to maintain and repair tissues,** as

well as, **manufacture hormones, enzymes, and other chemicals.**

- Proteins are made up of **amino acids,** of which the body normally manufactures 12.
- There are another 9 that must be obtained through food. These 9 amino acids are called **essential amino acids.**
- **Animal** proteins (meat and dairy) contain all essential amino acids and are called **complete proteins.**
- Some **plants** such as soy and buckwheat are, also, complete proteins.
- Other foods can be **combined** to form a complete protein, such as combining beans with rice or corn.
- **Recommended** protein intake varies depending on the size of the individual. It is usually recommended that adults consume 2-3 (4 oz) servings per day.
- **Examples of protein serving sizes are:** 1 egg, 1 ounce meat, or 1 tablespoon peanut butter.

Vegetables:

- This food group is **rich with vitamins and minerals.**
- Most of us could benefit by increasing our intake of vegetables.

- **Eat a variety** of vegetables to include the various vitamins and minerals, needed to stay healthy, i.e., **Vitamin A** is found in green vegetables, and **Vitamin C** is found in dark green and orange vegetables.
- **Recommended** daily intake is 2-3 servings. Eat a **variety of different vegetables** every week to meet bodily requirements for vitamins and minerals. Include **dark green and orange vegetables**, weekly.
- Since vegetables are **low in calories**, one can eat adequate amounts without the worry of gaining excess weight.

Fats:

- Provide **energy** to the body and **taste** to our foods.
- Assist in **growth and development**
- Aid in the **absorption of certain vitamins** into the body.
- Two major categories of dietary fats are **saturated** and **unsaturated**.
- **Saturated fats** are solid at room temperature, such as butter and shortening.
- **Unsaturated fats** are liquid oils, such as olive, vegetable, corn, and soybean oils.

- **Recommended: Limit** the use of **saturated fats**, which are associated with coronary artery disease.
- **Limit** use of **trans fats**, found in some margarines and processed foods, like crackers, cookies, and snack food.

Cholesterol:

- A **steroid** found in animal fats.
- An essential component of body **cell membranes.**
- Used for the manufacturing of **bile salts, steroid hormones, and Vitamin D.**
- Plays an important role in **cell transportation** and **nerve conduction.**
- Can be **detrimental when taken in high quantities,** especially in relation to heart disease.
- **Formed within the body**, which also, recycles it. Therefore, not dependent on the need to consume large quantities.
- **Foods** that contain cholesterol are **animal fats,** such as meats, egg yolks, and cheese.

Vitamins:

- Organic compounds that are **essential nutrients,** necessary to maintain good health.
- Some vitamins are **water soluble and** others are **fat soluble.**

- **Water soluble vitamins are:**
- **Dissolved** easily in water.
- Readily **excreted** from the body.
- **Daily intake** is needed.
- Water Soluble vitamins **include** the **Vitamin Bs,** such as Thiamin, Riboflavin, Niacin, Biotin, and Folic acid, **Vitamin B12,** and **Vitamin C.**
- **Fat soluble vitamins are:**
- **Absorbed** through the intestinal tract with help from fats in the diet.
- Tend to **accumulate** in the body and more likely to cause **overdoses.**
- Fat soluble vitamins **include** Vitamins **A, D, E, and K.**
- Eat a **varied diet** that includes fruits, vegetables, whole grains, and dairy products, to receive sufficient vitamins for good health.
- **Some medical conditions** may contribute to either vitamin accumulation or deficiency, such as pernicious anemia and malabsorption syndromes.

Dietary Minerals are:

- **Chemical elements** required by the body to carry on various crucial functions.
- Divided into two groups: **trace and macro** (major) minerals.

- These groups are identified based on the **daily amount** that is required by the body.

Trace elements:

- Small amounts required on a daily basis.
- Still important elements for body health.
- **Include** fluoride, iodine, iron, and zinc.

Major minerals:

- **Include** calcium, chlorine, magnesium, phosphorus, potassium, sodium, and sulfur.

Functions of minerals:

- Provide **structure.**
- Maintain **heart rhythm, muscle contractility,** conduction of **nerve impulses,** and **acid base balance**.
- Regulate **metabolism.**

Our bodies do not manufacture minerals, so we need a **daily intake** of these elements. On the other hand, we need to **avoid an excess** intake, which can lead to toxic effects. One common example of minerals in danger of excess intake is sodium and chloride, found in table salt.

The body functions to excrete excess amounts of minerals, but **some diseases** can lead to excess amounts of minerals and toxic effects. The **supplemental** intake of minerals is **discouraged,** except when ordered by a physician.

Some minerals are important enough to discuss in more detail. **Four important trace minerals** are fluoride, iodine, iron, and zinc.

Fluoride:

- Important for **dental** health.
- Also, important for healthy **bone** structure.
- **Sources** of fluoride include fluorinated water and fish bones.

Iodine:

- Important in the production of **thyroid hormones.**
- **Seafood** and ionized salt are good sources of iodine.

Before the 1950s, people with **goiters** (enlarged thyroid in the neck area) were relatively common in locations that did not have regular assess to seafood. Some people could develop a goiter because their thyroid overworked, due to **lack of iodine intake.** The problem was solved when iodine was added to table salt.

Iron:

- Important component of many body **enzymes**, such as **hemoglobin** and **some proteins**.
- Important for the **transportation of oxygen.**
- People **at risk** for low iron blood levels are **children, teens,** and **heavy menstruating women.**
- **High levels** of iron pose an increased risk for cardiac disorders and atherosclerosis (hardening of arteries).
- **Food sources** include liver, red meats, whole grains, and dark green vegetables.

Zinc:

- Important for the regulation of **metabolism, wound healing,** and **growth/development**.
- Some authorities question whether the intake of zinc **supplements** is beneficial.
- There is some concern supplements might be harmful, especially for the elderly.
- **Natural food sources** are always safer.
- **Food sources** are meat, liver, eggs, and oysters.

Important **macro minerals** include calcium, chloride, sodium, potassium, and phosphorus.

Calcium:

- **An electrolyte** that older people, especially women, need to include in their daily diet.
- Important for maintenance of **bone** health, and the functioning of **muscles and nerves.**
- There are many good **sources** for calcium, of which milk is the best.
- **Other sources** include cheese, ice cream, broccoli, salmon, and orange juice with added calcium and vitamin D.

Chloride:

- Along with sodium, it helps maintain body **fluid balance and acid-base balance.**
- **Food sources** are the same as sodium, such as table salt, processed foods, milk products, eggs, and seafood.

Sodium:

- Important for the maintenance of **fluid and acid-base balance.**
- **Food sources** are table salt, processed foods, milk, eggs, and seafood.
- **Excess sodium** can lead to high blood pressure and osteoporosis.

Potassium:

- An electrolyte important for **heart and nerve function.**
- Functions to maintain **muscle contraction** and normal **blood pressure**.
- Found in many **foods,** including fruits, vegetables, meats, and milk.

Phosphorus:

- An essential mineral in **bone formation and maintenance.**
- Important for **acid-base balance,** production of **energy,** and **nerve** function.
- **Food sources** are grains, meats, fish, milk products, and eggs.

Water:

- Essential for survival, since it is a crucial part of the **metabolic processes** of the body.
- Helps **flush toxins** from the body, **transport nutrients** to cells, **regulate body temperature, lubricate joints,** and provide a **moist** environment.
- **Recommendations** for daily intake of water varies. Water makes up about 70% of the body. Normally, we **tend to lose 2.5 liters per day.**

Under normal circumstances, one needs to replace what is lost to avoid dehydration. Six to eight cups of water daily is the general **recommendation**. Eight cups is equivalent to approximately 2 liters. Daily food intake provides another 0.5 liter.

The sensation of **thirst** reminds us to drink water, but most experts warn, that by the time we experience thirst, we are already dehydrated. In a healthy individual, there is little danger of over hydration because of the regulatory processes of the body.

Factors that influence the increase of fluid output include exercise, the environment, illness, and health conditions. Milk and juices are **good sources** of water but their sugar content tends to slow the rate of water absorption into the body's cells. . **Water is our best source** for fluid replacement.

We need to be careful about depending on **coffee and tea** for our main fluid intake, since they have dehydrating qualities. **Alcoholic** beverages, also, can be dehydrating.

There is a **close relationship** between our **fluid balance** and **electrolyte balance**. If we take in large quantities of water over a short period of time and it is not balanced with salt intake, the sodium chloride concentration can be diluted. Usually our body will **work to restore** the correct concentration. Someone who has impaired kidney function would have more difficulty restoring that balance.

Sport drinks help to provide replacement of water **and electrolytes,** when performing active exercise. However, we **need to be careful** not to overdo their intake, when not experiencing excess fluid loss.

Water is the best option for fluid replacement for moderate exercise (less than 1 hour). It is best to drink water while exercising so one does not become dehydrated in the first place. An advantage of sport drinks is because of the flavor: people will tend to drink them more than they will water. **Do not forget:** sport drinks contain electrolytes. **Flavored water would be a better option**.

For more specific information about nutrition, **My Pyramid (foodpyramid.com),** is an excellent site offered by the US Department of Agriculture (USDA). It provides basic information about the food groups and helps you work out an individualized food plan.

In 2011, the USDA changed **My Pyramid to My Plate (choosemyplate.gov),** in an effort to provide a chart that is easier for the average individual to understand and remember. The latest chart uses **a plate** to demonstrate recommended food proportions. **Recommendations** are that half your plate contains fruits and vegetables, with the emphasis on vegetables. The other half includes protein and grains. The diagram also includes a glass of dairy on the side.

CHAPTER VII

STAYING HEALTHY II

EXERCISE

Many studies about exercise show that it benefits senior citizens in many ways. Not only does **regular, moderate exercise** delay the onset of various illnesses and disabilities, but it can also improve those same conditions, if the individual already has them.

Regular exercise strengthens the **heart and lungs,** lowers **blood pressure**, strengthens **bones and muscles**, improves **balance** and joint **flexibility,** and controls **body weight**. It also improves **mental health:** we sleep better, we have improved self confidence, and it helps us stay socially active.

Additionally, exercise has been found to control and sometimes prevent **adult onset diabetes. Other diseases/ conditions** that can improve when one participates in regular exercise are heart disease, hypertension, stroke, arthritis, and osteoporosis.

Most authorities **recommend** 30 to 60 minutes of moderate exercise 2 to 4 times a week. The most important aspect is that it be done on a **regular basis**. If you are not used to regular exercise, you should start slowly. Begin with 5 to 10 minutes, twice a week, and then gradually increase the time.

Pay attention to what your body is telling you during exercise. If you experience pain or shortness of breath, stop or modify what you are doing. Don't forget to **consult your physician,** if you have a medical condition, **before beginning** an exercise program.

Some **recommended exercises** are walking, bike riding, water aerobics, swimming, or dancing. Most of these are **low impact** exercises that help protect your joints. It is important you choose something you enjoy. That will help you carry through on your program.

Pick a **time of day** that works best for you. I like to exercise early in the morning because I have found, that if I put it off, I end up not doing it. Some people like exercising alone, while others do better if they have a buddy or a group with whom to exercise. Other activities that help keep you socially and mentally active are bowling, nature walks, table games, crafts, gardening, crossword puzzles, reading, and volunteering.

MAINTENANCE OF MEMORY AND MENTAL ACTIVITY:

Mental competence is an important concern for senior citizens. Activities that involve healthy relationships. tend to maintain mental alertness best.

There are many **ways to participate** in healthy relationships, even if you do not have many family or friends close by.

Volunteering provides an opportunity for meaningful activities.

Many communities have **adult activity centers** available. For the disabled, there are **Adult Day Care** centers. **Assisted living facilities** provide a schedule of activities for their residents. **Mobile home parks for Seniors** usually provide an array of activities. Many communities, also, have various **social and recreational activities** available.

Additionally, give your **brain regular workouts** through memory activities, such as working puzzles and reading. Good **diet,** physical **exercise,** and good **sleep** habits are also important for maintaining brain health. We **don't know how** to completely prevent dementia or Alzheimer's Disease, but some of the activities, mentioned above, seem to help delay and slow the process.

REMINDER: Anything that gets you up, dressed, and out of the house on a regular basis is a good activity for physical and mental health.

ADDICTIVE BEHAVIOR:

There is an **increased concern** about addictive behavior among the senior citizen group. We used to believe that those over 65 years, who had problems with addiction, were people who always had addiction problems.

In recent years, healthcare professionals have been treating more seniors for addiction who had never demonstrated any signs of addiction before the age of 65. It is felt **factors that may trigger** addictive behavior in this age group are **major**

changes, such as loss of a spouse, friends or a pet, retirement, and/or loss of health of one's self or their spouse.

Common substances abused by the elderly are alcohol, prescription drugs (esp. tranquilizers & sedatives), and over the counter (OTC) medications. Older individuals are more prone to **experience increased intoxication** due to decreased metabolism, and reduced kidney and liver function, both of which occur with aging. Also, some tranquilizers have longer lasting effects in the elderly. The elder abuser frequently combines alcohol with other drugs, which intensifies the dangers.

Addictive behavior in the senior age group **frequently goes unnoticed** for several reasons. Often the individual lives alone. It is hard for family and friends to believe that Mom or Dad has a problem. Also, the signs may be mistakenly attributed to a medical condition, such as dementia, depression, or Parkinson's disease. Frequently, the abuser learns to avoid detection of multiple drug prescriptions by visiting several doctors and using different pharmacies.

Some **common signs** exhibited by someone who may be abusing substances are memory lapses, coordination problems, falls, bruises, irritability, depression, changes in sleeping, eating, and/or bathing habits, loss of interest in usual activities, and the tendency toward isolation.

What can be done about this problem?

- **Prevention** is always the best treatment.

- **Becoming aware** of the problem is a good first step.
- **Stay active** physically and socially.
- **Keep in touch** with family and friends.
- If concerned about an elder or yourself, the **family physician** is a good resource.
- Ask a **pharmacist** to run a drug interaction study of all of the individual's medications (prescription, OTC, and herbal).
- **Once you know** that substance abuse is a problem: **Encourage** medical and clinical treatment, including support group therapy.
- **Alcoholic's (www.aa.org) and Narcotic's Anonymous (www.na.org)** continue to be excellent resources.
- **ALANON (www.alanon.org)** is a good resource for family members and friends.

PREVENTIVE HEALTHCARE:

Is the major means for us to remain healthy and productive. Today we have more opportunities to **live longer and healthier** lives, but we do not always take advantage of those opportunities.

In the first part of the 20th century, people (mostly men) **smoked**, however, at that time they did not realize its dangers. Today, we **do know that smoking is dangerous,** but there are still many smokers. Sadly, some of these smokers are young people.

It is believed that people who have **high healthcare literacy** tend to live longer, healthier lives. Because they understand the benefits of preventive healthcare, they take advantage of the recommended **screening for cancer,** such as mammograms and colonoscopies. They are also more likely to have an annual health checkup and obtain regular flu and pneumonia **vaccinations.**

Medicare, Medicaid, and health insurance providers realize that **preventive healthcare** measures lead to **lower healthcare costs.** Therefore, they offer many of these preventive services for little or no cost to the patient.

The U.S. Department of Health and Human Services is concerned that a high percentage of Medicare recipients **do not take advantage** of preventive services. This seems to be, especially, true among minority groups. It is thought that many people do not take advantage of these services because they do not understand the importance, nor do they realize many of these services are covered by Medicare and other insurances.

Another reason people do not utilize these services is because they are **afraid** of discomfort or are afraid of receiving "bad news". However, if these procedures are avoided, there is a **greater chance** of receiving "bad news".

Those who remain current about health information can better understand what their doctors are telling them. Don't be afraid to ask your doctor questions. In fact, I encourage you to **write down your questions** so you don't forget them when you are with the doctor.

Don't feel intimidated about asking questions. You may feel the doctor is busy and you don't want to hold him or her up. Remember, that is their job. They depend on you to let them know what you do not understand.

Medicare offers a handbook named, **"Medicare & You"**, which discusses information about available Medicare services. If you no longer have that booklet, I suggest you send for a new copy and keep it handy, so you can refer to it from time to time.

SAFETY PRECAUTIONS:

Safety is more crucial for the older generation than for younger people because an injury can be more devastating and recovery may be slower and more difficult.

Fall Prevention, for the elderly, has become a number one concern of healthcare professionals. Fall prevention begins in the home. **A safe home** is more important for older citizens than for those under the age of 50, because older citizens tend to have poorer eyesight, hearing, balance, and strength.

Many people like having decorative **area rugs** around the house, but they can be a source for tripping or slipping. If you have an area rug that you do not want to dispose of, make it safer by taping it in place.

Good lighting is crucial, especially if the individual needs to get up in the middle of the night. Even surfaces are important, but not always practical. If you have any uneven areas, good lighting and handrails help.

Clear pathways are also important. Clutter not only contributes to the chance of falling, but it also contributes to fire hazards.

The **bathroom** seems to be the area where many accidents occur. **Handrails** help with getting in and out of the shower or bathtub and preventing slips and falls. **Nonskid** tubs or showers are important. **Shower/ tub chairs** help someone who experiences weakness or imbalance. **Chair height toilets** or a stool riser on the toilet helps someone who has trouble getting up and down.

Always wear **sturdy footwear,** even when getting up during the night. If you have problems with balance, **exercise** helps strengthen your muscles and improve balance. It is, also, wise to use a **cane** or a **walker,** if you are unsteady.

Older people, especially those who live alone, should seriously consider a **medical alert system**. My mother lived alone. One day she fell, broke her hip, and was not able to get to the phone to call for help. She laid on the floor for a couple of days before someone found her.

Once you get a medical alert device, you need to **wear it, all the time.** It does no good, if you don't have it on when you fall. Having someone check on you daily is helpful, but a medical alert system is a better option.

Besides considering home safety, **fire safety** and **security** against break-ins, also, need to be considered.

Fire Safety:

I've already mentioned the dangers of **clutter,** especially near an open flame, such as a pilot light.

Take precautions when **cooking** over an open flame. Probably one of the biggest dangers for senior citizens when cooking, is if they become **forgetful** and leave a cooking pot on the stove.

There are some people who think they can save money on **heating** by turning on their stoves to warm their homes. This can be a dangerous practice.

Senior citizens tend to experience poor circulation, which causes them to become chilled and have cold feet. They may use **space heaters** for warmth. They should never place their feet directly on the heater. If they have numbness in their feet, they will probably not be aware of an injury until it is too late.

A space heater should be kept at least **3 feet away** from curtains and papers. Space heaters should never be left on all night, nor when unattended.

It would be ideal if seniors **did not smoke**. However, if they do, they need to take the usual **precautions,** such as **never smoke in bed.** In addition, if they are exhibiting signs of forgetfulness, they should always be supervised when smoking.

Some people like the atmosphere of burning **scented candles,** but they still pose a fire hazard. Today, **battery powered candles** can provide the same ambiance as a burning candle, without the fire danger.

You always want to keep your home safe by making sure you have working **fire alarms.** Many people have fire alarms, but don't bother to make sure there are functioning batteries in them. The batteries need to be replaced at least once a year. A small **fire extinguisher,** in working condition, is handy to have, especially in the kitchen.

Have a **plan,** in case you have a fire. Once we had a garage fire. The fire marshal remarked that the reason the fire did not spread was because my husband **re-closed the door,** after he found the fire and then called 911. Whenever we go out of town, we always close all the bedroom doors, in case of a fire.

You should pre plan exits for everyone in the house, in case of fire. There should be at least **two exits.** When I was a home care nurse, I would always check the clients' homes for safety. It was surprising how many people would have one of their exits blocked with an appliance or a stack of boxes.

It is good, to occasionally, **practice** exiting the house, in case of an emergency. School children react best, in an emergency, because they are comfortable exiting their schools, due to repeated practice.

Home and Personal Security:

In addition to fire safety, **Home Security** from **Burglary and Scams** are also a concern for seniors. Statistics show they are, overall, less likely to be victims of crime, but seniors still feel vulnerable and need to take precautions.

Make sure you use **secure locks,** such as **bolt locks,** and actually use them. Be careful where you leave a spare key. The first place a thief looks for a key is under the door mat or a flower pot.

REMINDERS:

- Don't leave **windows** unlocked.
- Participate in **Neighborhood watches**.
- If a **stranger** comes to the door and claims to represent a particular company or agency, **ask for their ID.**
- If still unsure, **phone their company** before letting them in the house.
- **Security doors** are handy because you can see and speak with an individual who comes to the door while still keeping the door locked.
- Having a **home security system** is a good idea, especially if you live alone.

When **leaving your home**, take precautions. Women should always carry their **purses** close to their body. Men should always keep their **wallets** in a front inside pocket. Avoid carrying large amounts of cash. **Cell phones** are always helpful to have, in case of an emergency.

Do not leave your car unlocked.

When I was in my twenties, a friend and I stopped at a grocery store. Unwisely, we left the car unlocked, while we were gone. Unfortunately, we picked up an **uninvited passenger**. We didn't discover him right away. When he did pop up from the back seat, with his gun, it was on a well lit, busy street. This helped us feel brave enough to jump out of the car and get away. That was the last time that I left my car unlocked.

Be aware of your surroundings. If you notice someone or a group of individuals you think look suspicious, avoid them. They may be perfectly innocent, but why take the chance?

Probably the greatest criminal threats for Seniors are **fraud and con games.** Like the saying goes; "If it sounds too good to be true, it probably is".

Don't hesitate to say no, hang up the phone, or close the door. The older generations have been trained to be polite, but there is nothing impolite about saying no to someone who is trying to separate you from your money.

REMINDERS:

- **Don't give out** your name, address, credit card number, etc., to solicitors.
- Be aware of **home repair fraud,** which is a common scheme used on single elderly women.
- If the proposal being presented to you seems interesting, **get information in writing**.
- Put the individual off; tell them you want to **do further investigation** and then you will contact them.
- Today, we have easy access to useful resources, such as the **Better Business Bureau and the police**.
- If you are suspicious, be sure to **notify the police, company,** or **bank**, whichever is appropriate.

Driving Safety:

Another issue that faces Senior Citizens is: **WHEN IS IT NO LONGER SAFE TO DRIVE?**

This is a difficult issue for both the Senior and close family members. For the Senior, it represents a **loss of independence**. For **family members**, it is not easy "taking away the keys" when the Senior has always been their role model.

There are **different reasons** why someone is no longer a safe driver. These reasons include impaired sight or hearing, reduced flexibility or strength, reduced reaction time, and impaired judgment.

Some **early indications,** that there may be a concern about driving safety, are **"close call accidents ",** minor accidents (fender benders), scrapes from coming too close to a fence or mail box, **getting lost** in a commonly traveled area, and increased traffic **tickets or warnings.**

Some **resources** that may help in the decision making are the medical doctor, ophthalmologist or audiologist, and the motor vehicle department in your area. If you decide it would be safer to give up driving, there are some **resources** that can be utilized **for transportation**.

Once you adjust to the loss of driving, you may find you are **spending less money**. You no longer have to pay for gas, car maintenance, registration, and insurance. You may also find you are spending less money for cabs, bus or van service, than you did when maintaining a car. You might, also, end up getting **more exercise** walking or riding a bike.

This might be a good time to consider moving into a **senior living or assisted living facility,** that provides van service. Those facilities, also, offer a variety of activities which could expand your social contacts.

Frequently, communities have **shuttle services** available. In addition, you can, usually, find **delivery services** for groceries and pharmaceuticals.

If you are a **family member** of someone who has just given up driving, be sympathetic and realize the difficulty of adjusting to such a decision. **Be there** to help them adjust and offer transportation when you are able, or help find transportation alternatives.

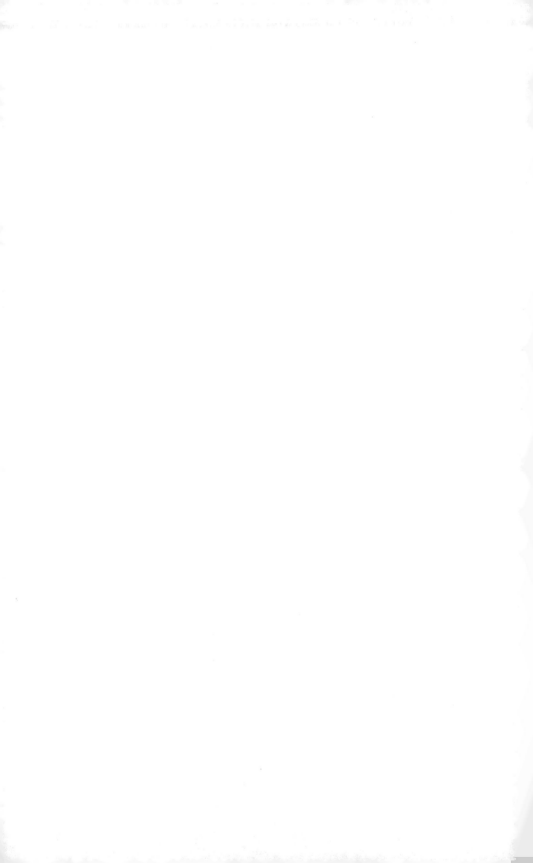

CHAPTER VIII

COMMON MEDICAL CONDITIONS I

Medical conditions can generally be divided into acute and chronic. **Acute** means a condition that develops rapidly. and usually has a short course. A **chronic** condition tends to develop over an extended period of time, and persists for a long time. Most chronic conditions can be controlled, but not, necessarily, cured.

The next two chapters are going to discuss a few conditions that are more prevalent for senior citizens, especially ones the individual can control with the help of healthcare professionals, and some that can be prevented.

ACUTE CONDITIONS:

Three acute conditions that senior citizens are more prone to experience and to develop more serious complications, than younger people, are the common cold, influenza, and pneumonia.

Common Cold:

Colds are usually experienced by all of us, one or two times each year. The cold is **caused** by a virus and usually runs a course of one to two weeks. If your symptoms persist beyond 2 weeks, you should see your primary care provider (PCP).

Usually, there is only a slight fever, but if you experience a high fever (103 or higher), you should see your PCP. Most often, the cold will run a mild course, but seniors, especially those with a chronic condition, need to be cautious and try to avoid exposure to colds, and care for themselves if they do get sick.

REMINDERS:

- Like most other conditions, the best **treatment** for the common cold is **prevention.**
- The number one preventive measure is **washing your hands**.
- Keep bathrooms and kitchens clean.
- Use clean glasses and eating utensils and do not share them.
- Steer clear of colds during cold season by **avoiding crowds** and people who have respiratory infections.

If you feel like you have a cold, avoid sharing it by **covering up when coughing or sneezing,** staying home when running a fever (even a low grade fever), and avoiding crowds. In addition to spreading through the air, the cold can spread by direct contact; therefore, avoid shaking hands and being in close contact with anyone, when you have a cold.

Since the cold is caused by a virus, there is **no known cure**, at least for the present time. **Antibiotics should not** be taken, unless ordered by the physician for a secondary bacterial infection.

However, there are measures which can be taken to **ease the symptoms.** First of all, get plenty of **rest** and drink lots of **fluids,** especially water.

Acetaminophen (Tylenol) can help for minor body aches. Be aware that acetaminophen can cause liver damage, if taken frequently, or in larger than recommended doses.

Take care in using decongestant nasal sprays, because they can cause a rebound effect. It is safer to use **saline nasal spray,** which helps to thin and loosen the accumulated mucus and moisten the airways.

Be aware that **cough and cold medicines** will not cure the cold any sooner. Be sure, if they are used, to read the instructions on the bottle carefully, including the side effects.

A **cold-mist humidifier** helps ease congestion and coughing. Everyone makes fun of the idea of taking **chicken soup** for colds or flu, but there seems to be some indication of symptom relief. There are, also, some people who feel they find relief of symptoms with the use of **Zinc, Vitamin C, and Echinacea.**

REMINDERS:

- **Avoid** spreading germs.
- **Cover up** when coughing or sneezing.

- **Wash hands**.
- **Dispose** of used tissues.

Influenza (Flu):

The flu is an infectious disease, caused by a virus. It is mainly spread through **air droplets**. It can, also, be transmitted by **direct contact** with objects that contain the virus.

Prevention:

It is possible for someone to pass on the flu virus before they, even, realize they are sick. Additionally, someone who is actively ill with the flu is contagious. Someone who **practices good hygiene,** such as consistent hand washing, is less likely to, inadvertently, expose someone else to the flu.

The **seriousness of a flu outbreak** will depend on the strength of the viral organism, if the flu vaccine matches the viral strain causing the flu, and the percentage of the population that has received the vaccine. When a high percentage of the population has received the flu shot for the season, there is less chance for the virus to spread.

A **yearly vaccination** is the most effective measure for prevention, especially for high risk individuals, including the elderly and those with compromising diseases, such as diabetes, heart disease, and chronic lung disease. Also, household members and caregivers of the high risk individuals should obtain vaccinations.

Most people can safely receive a flu shot, except those who are **allergic to chicken eggs,** have had a reaction to prior flu vaccinations, or have developed Guillain-Barre' syndrome from a previous flu shot. If you have a moderate or severe illness that involves a fever, it is recommended you wait to receive a vaccination until your symptoms cease.

Some **complications** of the flu are pneumonia, dehydration, and a worsening of some medical conditions, such as diabetes and heart disease. Like the **preventive precautions** for the common cold, the same precautions apply for Influenza.

Care for someone who has contacted the flu is similar to that of the common cold, except more so. First of all, **stay home,** especially when running a fever. Get plenty of **rest and drink** plenty of fluids, especially water. Try some chicken soup.

Contact your doctor if nausea, vomiting, or diarrhea persists, if symptoms continue beyond a week, or you are experiencing a high fever. Do not be afraid to be persistent with your physician, if one visit does not resolve the problem. Sometimes physicians get inundated with so many patients during cold and flu season, they may miss symptoms of a complication, like pneumonia. Of course, give the suggested treatment a couple of days to work.

REMINDERS:

- **Stay home** when sick.
- **Wash hands.**
- **Remember** to have an annual Influenza immunization.

Pneumonia:

Pneumonia is an inflammation of the lungs, due to an infection. It can be a complication from a different disease, such as a cold or flu. It can be caused by a virus or bacteria.

Antibiotics are effective if the organism is a bacteria, but not for a virus. When taking an antibiotic, be sure to **take the full course** ordered by the physician. Taking antibiotics unnecessarily or not completing the full course of therapy, contributes to the problem of antibiotic-resistant organisms.

The course for pneumonia can be mild to life threatening. The **degree of severity** depends upon the strength of the organism, the age of the individual, and the individual's immune system. People who have a high risk for pneumonia are those who have chronic lung disease, HIV/AIDS, heart disease, and smoke.

Signs and symptoms of Pneumonia include a persistent cough, chills and fever, shortness of breath, fatigue, and chest pain that fluctuates with breathing. Older people may experience a subnormal temperature, rather than a fever. If you experience these symptoms, you need to seek medical attention, as soon as possible, to avoid further complications.

The physician can determine the possibility of pneumonia by a direct physical examination. A chest x-ray can confirm its presence. Blood and mucus tests help determine the type of organism causing the illness.

The **treatment** includes taking the full course of prescribed medicine, and plenty of rest and fluids. It is important to return for any follow-up appointments. Pneumonia is a condition that can be prevented through receiving **seasonal flu shots,** a **pneumonia vaccination,** and keeping one's self healthy.

REMINDERS:

- **Avoid** indiscriminate use of antibiotics.
- Take **deep breaths and cough** to clear lungs.
- **Monitor** color and amount of sputum coughed up.
- **Report to physician**, if sputum becomes thicker and changes color, which becomes greener.
- Drink **fluids.**
- Do not forget to get a **pneumonia immunization.**

CHAPTER IX

COMMON CONDITIONS II

CHRONIC CONDITIONS
DIABETES MELLITUS (DM):
DM, more commonly known as Diabetes, is a chronic disease characterized by **impaired sugar metabolism.** This impairment is due to reduced insulin production, resistance to insulin by the body cells, or both. The decrease of sugar metabolism results in increased sugar in the blood, and lack of sugar utilization by the body for fuel and energy.

There are **three major types** of diabetes mellitus: **Type 1** (little or no insulin produced by the body), **Type 2** (impaired response to insulin), and **Gestational** diabetes (high blood glucose during pregnancy). This book will mainly discuss Type 2, since it is the most common one, and is usually the form that appears in adulthood.

Diabetes can be accompanied by many other **complications**. Two **acute complications,** that can be life threatening, are **hypoglycemia** (low blood sugar) and **hyperglycemia** (high blood sugar). Diabetes is associated with several **chronic complications,** including impairment of circulatory, cardiac, renal (kidneys), visual, and neurological systems. The better individuals regulate their diabetes, the better are their chances to avoid complications.

Risk factors include family history of diabetes, increase in age (45 years of **age** or older), and **obesity**. Additionally, national survey data indicates an increased risk for diabetes in certain **ethnic** groups, such as Native, Black, Hispanic, and Asian Americans.

People who are over 45 years of age should, periodically, have their blood sugar checked to make sure they are not developing diabetes. This is especially important, if they have a family history of diabetes, or have had gestational diabetes during pregnancy.

High blood sugar is a sign of Diabetes. Tests that help confirm a diagnosis of diabetes, include fasting blood glucose and glucose tolerance test.

Fasting blood sugar is considered indicative of a diagnosis of diabetes mellitus, when the results are higher than 126 mg/dl on two occasions. If an individual shows fasting levels between 100 and 126 mg/dl, they are considered to be **pre-diabetic**. It is estimated that there are many adults who are pre-diabetic, and have no idea they are at risk. A **normal fasting blood sugar** range for adults is 65-99 mg/dl.

A **glucose tolerance test** is a procedure that first measures the fasting blood sugar, to provide a baseline. Then the patient is given a high concentrated glucose drink. The blood glucose is then measured at predetermined intervals to assess how rapidly it returns to normal range. It should return to normal within 2 hours after ingestion of the glucose drink.

Another lab procedure used to diagnose diabetes and monitor how well individuals are managing their condition is **A1C**. It measures the average blood glucose for the previous 2-3 months. A **normal reading** for an A1C test is less than 5.7%. A reading for a **pre-diabetic** is between 5.7% to 6.4% and for a **diabetic** is 6.5% or above. The HbA1c is not used to replace daily blood sugar testing.

Classic **signs and symptoms** of diabetes are **excessive thirst** (polydipsia), **frequent urination** (polyuria), and **increased hunger** (polyphagia). These symptoms are related to the individual's high blood sugar. Other common symptoms include blurry vision, fatigue, and weight loss.

Treatment for diabetes involves medication, diet, exercise, and lifestyle modifications. The most important part of treatment involves education, because the management of diabetes involves so many basic aspects of one's life.

Most communities offer **Diabetic Education Programs,** especially for newly diagnosed patients. These programs utilize registered nurses and dietitians, to help patients learn to **manage their medications and diets.** Additionally, they learn about **complications** and ways to avoid them. These educational programs are, also, available for someone, who is not newly diagnosed, but may not have received sufficient information in the past, or has experienced changes in their condition.

Medications used for diabetes include **insulin** or a glucose lowering (**oral anti-diabetic**) medication. All individuals with **Type 1** diabetes need to take insulin, since their bodies are producing insufficient or no insulin at all.

Insulin is available in several different forms. There is **short acting, long acting, and a combination of the two.** Patients need information about the actions of the insulin type they are using. Insulin can be administered by a **syringe, pen, or pump.** The syringe is the most commonly used device, at this time.

Timing of the insulin injection with meals varies with the type of insulin being used. The goal is for the food sugar to reach the blood stream at the time insulin is working. For short acting insulin, it is important to **eat a meal** within 30 minutes after the injection. When taking a form of long acting insulin, it is important to have an **evening snack,** to maintain a safe blood glucose level during the night.

When **administering insulin**, make sure you measure the amount of insulin accurately. Also, accurate testing of your **blood sugar level** is important.

The **injection sites** need to be **rotated** to avoid formation of hard lumps or extra fatty deposits in the area. **Insulin can be injected** in the abdomen, arm, or thigh. Absorption at the abdominal site is faster, than the other two sites. It is best to use the same general area for injections, so the rate of absorption is the same with each shot.

When **checking** your **blood glucose**, first wash your hands. Prick the side of your finger with the lancet, to avoid sore spots on the tips of your fingers. There are many different glucose meters, so refer to the user manuals for operating instructions.

Strenuous exercise immediately after an injection can increase absorption. Regular exercise is good. Blood sugar levels need to be monitored closely, if engaging in more strenuous exercise than usual.

Alcohol use lowers blood glucose levels. One should always eat before, or while having an alcoholic drink. **Do not smoke** within 30 minutes of injection because it will interfere with the amount of insulin absorbed.

Be sure to wear a **medical alert ID,** at all times. Eat a carbohydrate if experiencing the **symptoms** of low blood glucose, such as hunger, trembling, sweating, rapid pulse, confusion, headache, nausea, or irritability.

Oral anti diabetic medications lower glucose blood levels in individuals with **type 2** diabetes. Ideally, people with type 2 diabetes would control their condition with **exercise and diet.** However, an anti diabetic medication may still be necessary, to assist with sugar utilization.

People who are taking these medications need to continue eating their **regular meals**, watch for **symptoms** of low blood sugar, monitor **blood sugar** levels, and carry **medical alert** identification. Always **carry candy** in case of low blood sugar episodes, and **avoid alcohol**. If the diabetic individual is **not responding,** it is a medical emergency, **CALL 911.**

A **well balanced diet** is the most important aspect of diabetic treatment. Many people, with type 2 diabetes, have been able to eliminate the need for medications and control their blood sugar levels by bringing their weight to normal levels.

The better individuals with diabetes maintain a balanced and nutritious diet, the greater is their ability to control their condition and avoid complications. A **goal of a balanced diet** for someone with diabetes is to keep blood glucose levels as close to normal as possible, which helps prevent or slow development of complications.

Diabetic diets are less stringent, today, than they used to be 15 or 20 years ago. Diabetic specialists realized that stringent diets tended to be counter productive for the diabetic individual.

If you need help to plan your meals, a **registered dietitian** is your best resource. **High fiber foods,** including vegetables and fruits, help to control your blood sugar level. **Avoid** eating sweets. **Fruits** provide a good substitute for sugared sweets.

Sugar substitutes are helpful, but still pay attention to the amount of calories in the low sugar foods you eat. Some people eat excess amounts of desserts, such as ice cream, because it is labeled low fat or low sugar. Do not assume you can eat as much as you want. Get into the habit of **checking labels** on all foods you purchase.

Try to keep your meals on a **regular schedule,** especially if you are taking insulin. In fact, people who maintain a regular schedule for their activities and sleep, usually are able to manage their condition better.

There are many **resources** for guidance, when planning meals for people with diabetes. The **American Diabetes Association (www.diabetes.org)** is probably the "number one" agency for help to deal with all aspects of diabetes. Another resource for nutritional guidance is the **US Department of Agriculture (www.usda.gov).**

Regular exercise is an important component of diabetic treatment, since it helps in the control of blood sugar, weight, and blood pressure. It is important to **consult your physician** before beginning an exercise program, especially if you have a heart condition. Your physician may have to adjust your medications depending on the effects of exercise on your condition.

It is best to try to exercise on a **daily basis** and be sure to wear protective footwear, drink plenty of water, and carry some fast acting carbohydrate food with you, in case you experience an episode of low blood sugar. **Lifestyle modifications** are necessary to regulate the diabetic condition and prevent complications.

Foot care is not always emphasized enough as part of diabetic care. People with diabetes often experience impaired circulation and increased numbness in their lower extremities. Frequently, someone with diabetes can have a small cut on the foot and are not aware of it, until it becomes infected. Lower extremity amputations are, unfortunately, common with diabetics.

First of all, wearing **protective footwear** that covers the foot is crucial. **Never** walk around in your **bare feet**. Some people who have stepped on a stone or pin may never realized it. Make sure that shoes are the right size. **Cotton socks** are best because they absorb moisture.

Wash your feet on a **daily** basis. **Inspect** them for redness, sores, blisters, or cuts. Take care when **trimming toe nails**. **Podiatry care** is recommended. Many insurances and Medicare will help pay for podiatry care for someone with impaired circulation.

REMINDERS:

- Since there are many serious complications associated with diabetes, it is important you **keep all medical appointments**.
- Test your blood sugar, as instructed by the physician, and **keep a log** of the results to take with you to your appointments.
- Keep track of any **low blood sugar episodes**, even mild ones, and record them in your log.
- **Notify** your healthcare provider if:
  Diet is not tolerated.
  Any nausea or vomiting.
  Any signs or symptoms of low or high blood sugars.

ARTHRITIS:

Arthritis is an inflammation of one or more joints of the body. There are several types of arthritis. The most common form is **Osteoarthritis** followed by **Rheumatoid arthritis (RA)**. **Osteoarthritis** is caused by either wear and tear on the joint, infection, or injury. **Rheumatoid arthritis** is an autoimmune disease. (Autoimmune conditions are ones where the body's immune system turns against the body.)

Osteoarthritis, which is associated with aging, can involve any joint but tends to involve the weight bearing joints, such as the back and hips. **Rheumatoid arthritis** is a systemic disease, which means it can affect other parts of the body, in addition to the joints. It tends to be symmetrical, which means it affects joints on both sides of the body. It involves all joints, including fingers, wrists, and knees.

Diagnosis of arthritis is made based on a physical examination, as well as, laboratory and radiology tests. **Symptoms** result from the breakdown of cartilage, which protects the joints. As the cartilage deteriorates, bone begins to rub against bone causing pain, swelling, and stiffness. As these symptoms progress, eventually the individual can become disabled.

The symptoms are generally worse in the morning. A **warm shower** helps provide relief of stiffness and pain. Unfortunately, there is **no cure** for arthritis at this time.

Depending upon the amount of discomfort and disability, physical and occupational therapy may be called for to assist the individual. **Physical therapy (PT)** provides exercises, including range of motion, to maintain and improve joint function and muscle strength. **Occupational therapy (OT)** provides help learning ways to reduce joint stress, when performing activities of daily living. OT and PT, also, provide **assistive devices** to help with activities and reduce joint stress. Examples of assistive devices include a cane, long handled pickups, or grab bars.

Medications can help provide comfort. The use of over-the-counter (OTC) medications is more desirable for the person with osteoarthritis, because there are fewer severe side effects.

Acetaminophen (Tylenol) is one OTC medication recommended for osteoarthritis. Liver damage is a concern, if Acetaminophen is taken with alcohol, or if more than the recommended dose is taken.

Non steroid anti-inflammatory drugs (NSAID), such as aspirin, ibuprofen (Advil, Motrin), Celebrex, or naproxen (Aleve), are more effective for inflammatory types of arthritis, such as Rheumatoid. Unfortunately, there are side effects when used long-term. These side effects include heart disease, stroke, kidney disease, gastrointestinal ulcers, inflammations, and bleeding disorders. Because of these side effects, it is important your healthcare provider knows you are taking these medications. Always, follow the recommended instructions for their use.

Many individuals with arthritis, especially the osteoarthritis type, function very well if they keep their **weight under control**, participate in **regular, moderate exercise,** and use over the counter **medications in moderation. Heat, ice and topical analgesic creams/ointments** have proven helpful for temporary joint pain relief.

If over-the-counter drugs are not effective, there are various prescription medications that the doctor might prescribe to improve the individual's quality of life. **Antirheumatic drugs** include methotrexate and gold salts.

Corticosteroids are, also, useful in the treatment of inflammatory joints. Many of these drugs do **modify the immune system,** so it is important you visit your doctor regularly. Individuals, taking these drugs, are at higher risk for **infections**. They need to take precautions to **avoid colds and flu** by avoiding crowds, staying away from ill people, and washing their hands frequently.

Some of these medications, such as corticosteroids, need to be **discontinued if** the individual is scheduled for **surgery** to insure wound healing and avoid wound infection. **Avoid abrupt discontinuance** of these drugs, especially the corticosteroids. Discontinuance of these drugs should always be done under medical supervision.

In recent years, a **new class of drugs** has been developed for rheumatoid arthritis called Biologic drugs. One such drug is **Humira**. These drugs are genetically engineered proteins, that have been derived from human proteins. They are designed to target specific parts of the immune system, rather than the entire system. These drugs appear to be more effective in relieving pain and slowing joint destruction.

A **disadvantage,** at this time, is that these drugs have to be injected, but drug companies are working to develop an oral form. These drugs have proven to be so successful that healthcare providers are starting to see the benefits of beginning drug treatment early, in order to prevent or delay joint damage. Frequently, these drugs will be given in combination with other antiarthritic medications.

Be careful about **quacks, gimmicks,** and treatments that claim to cure arthritis. Like the saying goes, "if it sounds too good to be true; it probably is". Some of these treatments are dangerous; others may not be dangerous, but do waste money. Your best bet is to consult your healthcare provider, preferably one who specializes in arthritis.

There are some **herbals,** such as Glucosamine/chondroitin, that are promoted for joint protection. Studies have not proven these are any more effective than a placebo, but they do not seem to be harmful for someone who appears to find relief by using them. It is still important that physicians know when a patient is taking any herbs.

Joint replacement surgeries have been a godsend for people with arthritis. When joint replacement surgeries were first being performed in the 1960s, people who had been in a wheelchair for years were able to walk again. To them it was like a miracle. Significant progress continues to be made with these procedures.

The **two major joint replacement** procedures, being performed, are for the hip and the knees. Most individuals who are experiencing unrelieved pain and difficulty performing common activities of daily living will benefit from these procedures.

In the 1960s, when these procedures were first being performed, the specialists were not sure how long the joint would last, or if there would be any unforeseen complications. Therefore, these surgeries were limited to people, who were 60 years or older. Since then, these surgeries have been so successful, younger people are now provided this option.

A **modified version** of the hip replacement is used for people with hip fractures, especially for the elderly. Those individuals are now able to recover more rapidly and avoid life threatening complications, such as pneumonia.

Orthopedic surgeons, who perform joint replacements, will caution that most people who undergo these procedures will usually experience improvement in mobility, but **should not** expect to **perform high impact activities,** such as jogging. These activities will increase joint wear and tear, and cause loosening of the joint.

Over the years, there was expected to be some wear on the joint and possibly loosening. However, the original surgeons who developed the joint procedures were surprised at how well these joints have lasted.

Specific preparations for joint surgeries include **auto blood donation,** that can be used for the surgery to reduce the risks associated with receiving blood from others. If any **other chronic diseases** exist, the physicians will want to ensure that these other conditions are stabilized. If individuals are **overweight**, they will be encouraged to achieve a safer weight level. Overweight people exert more pressure on the artificial joint, which can cause damage and loosening.

Infection of the joint is a **serious complication.** However, with appropriate precautions, occurrence of this complication is very low. Before surgery, you will be required to **bathe. Notify the surgeon** if there is any infection or rash present.

Many joint infections are related to an existing **urinary tract or dental infection.** Surgical preparation will include urinary tract and dental evaluations. Because of this ongoing risk, anyone with a joint replacement will need to notify their dentist of the procedure and take a **prophylactic antibiotic,** before they have any **dental work or other invasive procedures** performed. Routine teeth cleaning will be delayed for several weeks after the surgery.

Immediately following joint replacement surgery, pain medication is provided to keep the patient comfortable. Following a hip replacement, a **V-shaped pillow** will be placed between the legs to keep the hip in alignment and prevent hip dislocation.

Surgeons will frequently order a **continuous passive motion (CPM)** exercise machine for the patient who has had a knee replacement. This device is used to restore movement, decrease swelling by elevating the leg, and improve circulation through leg and joint motion.

Most patients will begin walking shortly after surgery, with the support of a walking aid and hospital staff member. **Physical therapy** will continue working with the patients until they can independently manage their exercises and function by themselves at home.

Hospitals used to keep joint replacement patients in bed longer, following surgery. However, it was observed that patients actually progressed faster and had less complications, such as pneumonia and blood clots, when they got up and around earlier in their recovery.

Blood clots in the leg are a concern with joint replacements, during the first several weeks. The surgeon will prescribe medications (blood thinners) and other measures to prevent clotting. Some of the measures include **support hose**, **inflatable leg coverings,** and **foot/ankle exercises**. **Symptoms** of a clot are pain, redness, and swelling in the calf or leg. If the clot spreads to the lungs, there will be shortness of breath and chest pain.

Wound care is important to prevent infection and promote healing. The sutures or staples will be removed approximately two weeks after surgery. Until the wound is healed, the patient needs to avoid getting it wet. A plastic dressing can be used to protect it while bathing.

When preparing for surgery, the patient will be evaluated as to how appropriate the **home environment** will be after surgery. The patient will need some assistance at home with bathing, cooking, shopping, and laundry, for several weeks.

Anyone, who does not have help available at home, will be advised to stay, for a short time, in an **extended-care or rehabilitation facility**. Medicare and secondary insurances will cover the stay as long as skilled care, such as physical therapy, is required.

Home modifications will probably be required to prevent falls and excessive bending at the hips (for hip surgery), **such as:**

- **Sturdy handrails** in the bath or shower
- **Sturdy handrails** in the stairways
- **Raised toilet seat**
- **Stable** shower or tub **bench**
- **Long-handled** bath sponge and shower hose
- **Dressing stick**
- **Sock application aid**
- **Long-handled shoe horn**
- **Reacher stick** for picking up items
- **Loose** electrical cords and rugs removed

Also, patients will need to use a **stable chair** with a firm back and two arms, to assist when standing and sitting. When sitting in the chair, the patient's knees should be lower than the hips, for those who have had hip replacement surgery. Knee replacement patients should have a **foot stool** for intermittent leg elevation.

Home care services are highly recommended, when patients first come home from the hospital or extended-care facility. The home care therapist will **evaluate the home situation**

and make any recommendations to help patients adapt, safely. to their new joint.

Not only will the therapist help patients with **learning exercises,** but will, also, help them learn **how to** get in and out of the shower, dress, climb stairs, get in and out of the car, and carry out other activities, without causing damage to their new joint. **If the bedroom is on an upper floor**, the surgeon may recommend that the patient sleep on the ground floor for a few weeks, until the joint has had a chance to heal, especially knee replacement patients.

The **success** of joint replacements **depends upon** how well the surgeon's instructions are followed. The patient's **activity program** includes a graduated walking program, along with specific exercises designed to restore movement and strength. These activities need to be performed several times, daily.

To **prevent dislocation** of the hip after a hip replacement, patients will be instructed not to cross their legs or bend their hips more than 90 degrees (right angle). Additionally, they need to avoid turning feet excessively in or out and to use a pillow between their legs when sleeping.

REMINDERS:

- Coordinate **pain medications** with activities.
- Avoid excess **joint stress**.
- Avoid extreme **environmental temperatures** and damp, moist environments.

- Avoid **stressful** situations.
- Avoid **sudden movements**.
- Allow **plenty of time** to perform activities.
- Resume **routine, low impact exercise,** when approved by the surgeon.
- **Water aerobics** is an excellent example of low impact exercise.
- Use correct **body alignment and mechanics** when lifting, reaching, bending, and walking.
- Use appropriate **assistive and supportive devices,** such as grab bars, toilet risers, canes, long-handled pickups, and braces.
- **Velcro closures** and zippers for clothing can be helpful.
- Maintain a **safe environment** by keeping clear pathways, night lights, and wearing well-fitting, sturdy shoes.
- Do not resume driving until **approved by** the surgeon.
- Become familiar with the **Arthritis Foundation** and what they have to offer (**www.arthritis.org**).
- The **American Association of Orthopedic Surgeons (AAOS)** web site has helpful information about joint replacements (**www.aaos.org**).

CHRONIC OBSTRUCTIVE LUNG DISEASE (COLD) or CHRONIC OBSTRUCTIVE PULMONARY DISEASE (COPD):

COPD is a disease characterized by an obstruction of the air flow in and out of the lungs and loss of lung elasticity. This condition is associated with chronic bronchitis, asthma, and emphysema. The lungs are the organs that transfer the oxygen in the air into the blood stream, in exchange for carbon dioxide to be expelled from the body.

Symptoms of COPD include shortness of breath, cough, and sputum production. The shortness of breath is associated with exercise in the early stages of the disease, but as the condition progresses, it is present even at rest.

At this time, there is no cure and the condition will progress. **Medical treatment** aims to slow the progression and help the patient to be active and function as well as possible. As with many chronic diseases, the best treatment is prevention.

Additional symptoms include wheezing, chest tightness, and tiredness. Symptoms of advanced COPD include weight loss, lung hypertension, heart failure, osteoporosis, heart disease, muscle wasting, and depression. Symptoms worsen with exposure to air pollutants and infections.

The **main risk factor** for COPD is **smoking**. The most important factor for slowing the progression of the disease is to completely stop smoking. There are some **occupational exposures**, such as mining and welding, associated with COPD, but these factors seem to be less significant than smoking.

Because of the **restricted airflow**, the person with COPD may not be able to completely finish exhaling before they need to inhale again. This leaves some excess air in the lungs. Additionally, there is a loss of lung surface area for exchange of oxygen and carbon dioxide (CO_2), which leaves **higher levels of CO_2** in the blood.

The **diagnosis** of COPD cannot be made by merely observing the individual's symptoms because there are other conditions that have similar symptoms. The various tests used to diagnose and monitor COPD include:

- **Pulmonary function tests** are done to confirm COPD.
- **Spirometry** is used to measure forced exhaled volume.
- The severity of the disease is measured based on shortness of breath severity and the amount of exercise limitation.
- **Chest x-rays** show over expanded lungs, a flat diaphragm, and increased airspace.
- Blood samples are used to study **arterial blood gases** (artery blood). (COPD patients will have low oxygen and high carbon dioxide levels in their blood.)

There is **no cure** for COPD, but it is preventable and treatable. As mentioned before, smoking is the main cause of COPD.

If you are a smoker, do anything you can to stop. It is hard, but **keep trying.** If you fail, even several times, keep trying. There are several programs for **smoking cessation** available. Some resources include local health departments, state departments of health services, local medical centers, and the **American Lung Association (www.lung.org)**.

There are also medications that can used in conjunction with these smoking cessation programs. The sooner you are able to stop smoking the better. Even when you are not completely successful in quitting, you are cutting down on your smoking.

Once COPD has been diagnosed, your healthcare provider can monitor your condition and order supportive treatments and medications. There are excellent **support programs and groups** that help individuals live with COPD. Your local medical center or health department can help you find a support group in your area.

Some of the current **medications** used for COPD are **bronchodilators,** that are inhaled to improve the airway flow. The bronchodilators do not slow the progression of the disease, but they can help improve the quality of life.

Another type of drug used is an **anticholinergic** that also helps to improve airway flow. There are **serious side effects** with these drugs, such as cardiac problems, therefore, close medical supervision is required.

Corticosteriods are also used for COPD to reduce inflammation of the airways. They, also, have **serious**

side effects and require close medical supervision. Corticosteriods should **never be discontinued abruptly** by the patient.

Supplemental **oxygen therapy** plays a major role in the treatment of COPD. People with COPD, who have low blood oxygen levels, benefit from a therapy of low concentrated oxygen. This therapy improves their exercise and activity levels, but it does not necessarily improve their shortness of breath.

Individuals need to be **cautious** to always keep the oxygen delivery at low rates. High concentrations of oxygen can cause a chronic accumulation of carbon dioxide that could eventually lead to respiratory failure.

Another **safety issue** for someone receiving continuous oxygen is **smoking**. Since oxygen supports combustion, there is always a **danger of fire** when someone smokes around an individual who is receiving oxygen.

Oxygen can be delivered by cylinder or a concentrator. A concentrator requires electricity so, if there is a power outage, oxygen cylinders are needed until the electricity becomes available again.

Pulmonary rehabilitation for COPD patients include a program of exercises, under the supervision of a pulmonary specialist, to help improve breathing and exercise tolerance. Those who are overweight are encouraged to lose weight, and those who are underweight are helped by an increase of their calorie intake.

REMINDERS:

- Use relaxation exercises during periods of shortness of breath.
- Avoid stressful situations and excessive exercise.
- Avoid medications and drugs that depress breathing, such as sedatives.
- Seek out help from a healthcare professional if experiencing depression.
- Drink plenty of fluids based on recommendations from your healthcare provider.
- Perform deep breathing exercises throughout the day.
- Pursing the lips when breathing out facilitates exhalation.
- Use of a wedge to elevate the upper body helps to ease breathing and promote chest expansion when lying in bed.
- With severe shortness of breath, sit up, lean forward, and support head and arms on a table with a pillow. (This position helps provide maximum chest expansion.)
- Wear or carry a medical ID card, tag, or bracelet.
- The American Lung Association (www.lung.org) is an excellent resource.
- Report any increased difficulty of breathing, or changes in color of sputum to healthcare provider.

- **Pace activities** with rest periods.
- Use **oxygen** during activities as appropriate.
- Use **energy-saving** devices and aids.
- **Build endurance** by increasing activities, every few days.
- **Prevent infections** by avoiding crowds and people who are sick, and always wash hands.
- If still **smoking,** keep trying to **QUIT**.
- Find a COPD **support group** to visit.

CHAPTER X

COMMON CONDITIONS III

CHRONIC CONDITIONS (cont.)
CHRONIC CARDIAC DISEASES:

There are some conditions that are called acute, such as an Acute Myocardial Infarction (heart attack), but are in fact related to a chronic condition. The symptoms may appear rapidly, but the causes of the episode have been present for a long time.

MYOCARDIAL INFARCTION (MI):

The MI, commonly known as a **heart attack,** involves an interruption in blood flow to the heart muscle, leading to the death of some of that muscle. This interruption in flow usually occurs when fatty plaques break off into the blood stream and become lodged in a cardiac artery.

The **classic symptoms** include chest pain radiating to the left arm, shortness of breath, weakness, indigestion, and fatigue. Although these are the classic symptoms, not everyone experiences them.

Chest pain can be a symptom of several medical conditions, but because of the life threatening nature of an MI, one should have **medical attention immediately,** when experiencing chest pain. If it turns out the cause was not an MI, there may not be an emergency, however, chest pain still indicates there is a condition which probably needs treatment.

Not everyone experiences chest pain when they are having a heart attack. **Women** tend to experience less typical symptoms. They are more likely to experience shortness of breath, fatigue, and indigestion. It is not unusual for the doctor to evaluate the woman for gall bladder disease when they are actually experiencing an MI. Other people may be experiencing **pain on the left side of the jaw,** which may be mistaken for a dental problem.

The chest pain is often described as a **pressure or tightness.** Some people describe it as feeling like "an elephant sitting on their chest". **Other symptoms** associated with an MI include nausea, vomiting, sweating, anxiety, and palpitations (rapid or irregular heart rate).

Risk factors include:

- family history
- previous heart attack
- diabetes
- smoking
- obesity
- chronic kidney disease
- high blood levels of certain lipids and cholesterol
- high blood pressure
- chronic high stress level

- alcohol abuse
- drug abuse, especially cocaine and methamphetamine
- People with any of these risk factors should be on the alert for the possibility of a heart attack.

Diagnosis is made based on symptoms, medical history, electrocardiogram (ECG/EKG), coronary angiogram, and laboratory studies.

Immediate treatment includes aspirin, nitroglycerin, and oxygen. Some victims benefit from thrombolysis therapy, which dissolves the clot blocking the artery.

Cardiac catheterizations are done to identify the vessels that are affected and the percentage of blockage. A **stent or bypass surgery** may be appropriate, depending on the findings.

The damaged heart tissue conducts electrical impulses more slowly, which can cause a lethal **arrhythmia** (abnormal heart rhythm). The most lethal arrhythmia is ventricular fibrillation (fast, chaotic heart beat), which needs cardiac defibrillation to terminate the abnormal rhythm.

Prevention is provided through a **healthy lifestyle,** including regular exercise, normal body weight, and a healthy diet. **In addition,** patients should avoid smoking, limit alcohol intake, control blood pressure, and follow treatment for other underlying conditions, such as diabetes.

REMINDERS:

- Follow instructions regarding **medications** and report any side effects.
- Report any **pain**.
- Keep **emergency phone numbers** available.
- Gradually increase **daily exercise** program.
- **Rest** before and after exercising.
- **Avoid** stress, heavy meals, heavy lifting, caffeine, other stimulants, and extremes in temperatures.
- **Cease activity and call medical provider** if experiencing symptoms of intolerance, such as pain or shortness of breath.
- Seek out **cardiac rehabilitation** programs and support groups.
- **Monitor** pulse and blood pressure, record and report these at medical appointments.
- Rest before **sexual activity**.
- **Consult medical provider** about any recommended precautions related to sexual activity.
- **Avoid straining** with bowel movements.
- Carry **medical identification**.
- Use the **American Heart Association (www.heart. org)** for support and literature.

CONGESTIVE HEART FAILURE (CHF):

CHF is a condition in which the heart is unable to pump sufficient blood supply to meet the needs of the body.

There are several **risk factors** that can lead to this condition. **Diseases** that impair the pumping action of the heart comprise the most common risk factors. Some of these diseases are hypertension, coronary artery disease, heart valve disease, and alcohol abuse. Less common factors are thyroid and heart rhythm disorders.

There are also some **medications** taken by individuals with heart disease that can cause salt retention or affect the heart muscle. Some examples include:

- Nonsteroidal anti-inflammatory drugs (NSAID), such as ibuprofen (Motrin) and naproxen (Aleve)
- Some oral diabetic medications (Avandia or Actos)
- Some calcium channel blockers

This information emphasizes the importance of keeping **regular contact** with your healthcare providers. Some **other major risk factors,** not mentioned above, are smoking, obesity, and diabetes.

Symptoms of CHF vary depending on the side of the heart that is impaired, and the risk factors contributing to the disorder. The **most common** symptoms are shortness of breath, diminished exercise tolerance, fatigue, and swelling of the legs.

If the impairment of the pumping action is **on the left side** of the heart, the lungs tend to be affected first, because the heart cannot handle all the blood **returning from the**

lungs. Shortness of breath and accumulation of fluid in the lungs becomes apparent.

If **the right side** of the heart is affected, it has a hard time handling the blood **returning from the body** and tends to exhibit swelling in the lower extremities. Untreated left-sided failure can lead to right-sided failure, so the individual will end up with symptoms described for failure of **both sides**.

Diagnosis is made using medical history, physical examination, chest x-ray, ultrasound, and laboratory tests. A **chest x-ray and ultrasound** will show an enlarged heart, and the amount of blood the heart is able to eject with each beat. **Electrocardiograms (EKG)** will show arrhythmia's (abnormal heart rhythms) and other abnormalities associated with heart failure.

Of course, **prevention** is the **best treatment** for any chronic condition. The best way to prevent CHF is to control the risk factors. **Lifestyle changes** are probably not the easiest things to do, but can be the most effective. The sooner the changes are made, the better.

Anyone with a **family history** of heart disease, hypertension, diabetes, or already has one or more of these diseases, should definitely **make changes.** Helpful changes include moderate exercise, weight reduction, smoking cessation, decrease of alcohol intake, reduction of salt intake, stress management, blood pressure control, and limitation of cholesterol and saturated fat intake.

If you already have one of the diseases associated with CHF, be sure to take prescribed medications, keep medical appointments, and follow medical advice. Chronic disease management involves medication therapy, lifestyle modification, and control of the underlying disease. An implanted defibrillator and heart transplant may be options for severe cases.

REMINDERS:

- **Avoid fatigue** by alternating rest periods with activities.
- **Sleep** with head elevated via a wedge pillow to ease shortness of breath and   improve rest.
- Do not take any **over-the-counter drugs** without authorization from primary medical provider.
- Pay attention to **precautions** regarding medications and report any adverse reactions.
- **Report** any increase in symptoms, such as fatigue, shortness of breath, coughing, anxiety, or leg swelling.
- **Weigh** yourself, as instructed, using the same scale, same amount of clothing, and first thing in the morning.
- **Avoid strenuous** activity and exercise.
- **Carry** medical identification information.

CEREBROVASCULAR ACCIDENTS (CVA):

A CVA, commonly known as a **Stroke,** is an interruption of the blood flow to a part of the brain. It is the third leading cause of death and the first leading cause of long-term disability in the US.

There are two main **types of strokes. Ischemic** is the most common type and occurs when there is a restriction of blood flow within a vessel that provides blood supply to the brain. This type may be due to a narrowing of the vessel or a blockage caused by a clot.

The second most common type is **hemorrhagic,** which occurs when a blood vessel within the brain weakens and bursts. When the blood flow is interrupted, brain cell damage and cell death will begin to occur within minutes. Damaged brain cells cannot be regenerated.

It is essential that the victim is **treated immediately** to minimize the damage. The goal is to restore blood flow and oxygen as soon as possible. Individuals experiencing **hemorrhagic strokes** may benefit from **neurosurgery**.

A victim with an **ischemic stroke** may be treated with a **thrombolysis drug** (clot buster), if seen within 3 hours of onset of symptoms, but unfortunately, most people do not get to the hospital rapidly enough for the treatment. Not only is it important to get to the hospital immediately after symptoms appear, but also, be sure to communicate the problem to the ER personnel so they can act immediately. This is one time that the use of **911** could facilitate rapid attention for the victim.

Diagnosis is made based on symptoms, medical and family history, and diagnostic tests. Also, Computed Tomography (CAT scans), Electroencephalograms (EEG), and spinal taps are frequently used.

The resulting symptoms depend upon the part of the brain that is affected. The **main symptoms** include inability to move one or both limbs on one side of the body, inability to understand language or to speak, and/or inability to see one side of the visual field.

Other physical symptoms include muscle weakness, numbness, headaches, pressure sores, pneumonia, incontinence, and slurred or loss of speech. **Emotional symptoms** may occur, such as anxiety, apathy, depression, and emotions (laugh, cry) that don't match the occasion. **Cognitive symptoms** include disorders involving perceptions, speech, and memory.

The **initial symptoms** of a stroke tend to come on suddenly. Some people experience **TIAs (transient ischemic attacks)** which are like mini strokes. Early treatment of a TIA could prevent the occurrence of a major stroke.

Treatment to recover from lost function involves the use of a **multidisciplinary rehabilitation team** involving nursing, physical therapy, occupational therapy, and speech-language therapy. **Rehabilitation** for the stroke victim needs to begin immediately.

Nursing care works to maintain skin integrity, nourishment, hydration, and prevent disabilities through proper positioning. Nursing care also prevents other complications by monitoring vital signs, levels of consciousness, respiratory capacity, and cardiac status.

Physical and occupational therapy tend to overlap. **Physical therapy** tends to manage range of motion of the joints, muscle strength, ambulating (walking), sitting, and standing. **Occupational therapy** works on activities of daily living (eating, bathing, dressing, cooking, etc.) and other occupational activities. **Speech-language therapy** works with speech, reading, and swallowing.

Most **function** that is going to return will occur within the first few months of rehabilitation, but victims will continue to show improvement for years. Results depend on the amount of damage, how soon therapy is started, and the motivation of the patient.

Medical treatment includes control of high blood pressure, medications to reduce blood cholesterol, and blood thinners. Laboratory tests will be used to monitor cholesterol, bleeding, and clotting times.

Risk factors for a stroke include older age, high blood pressure, high cholesterol, previous stroke, diabetes, heart arrhythmias, smoking, drug use, and heavy alcohol use. The illegal drugs commonly associated with stroke are cocaine and amphetamines.

REMINDERS:

- **Follow** medical, nursing, and therapy **instructions** regarding **exercises**, positioning, support of limbs, safety precautions, and **medication** administration.
- **Keep appointments** with all rehabilitation professionals.
- **Use assistive aids/devices,** as needed, to perform activities of daily living.
- **Adjust home environment** to improve safety and accommodate wheelchair or other assistive aids.
- **Avoid constipation** through increased fluid intake, increased bulk in the diet, and increased exercise/activity.
- **Monitor vital signs** and report to healthcare professional.
- **Make lifestyle changes,** as appropriate, by losing weight, controlling blood pressure, stop smoking, stop illegal drug use, and avoid excess alcohol use.
- If taking blood thinners, **watch for signs** of bleeding and bruising.
- **If difficulty swallowing,** Eat small amounts of textured and thickened foods.
- Place foods on unaffected side of mouth and allow plenty of time to chew and swallow food.
- Avoid milk and thin, smooth foods.

- Utilize the **American Stroke Association** as a useful resource (www.strokeassociation.org).
- **Report** any emotional deficits, such as depression, confusion, or memory loss.
- **Utilize** community, social services, and psychological support agencies, as appropriate.

DEMENTIA:

Dementia is a **loss of cognitive ability** which can include memory, problem solving, attention, and language, which exists **for 6 months or more**. There are **several types and causes,** but the most common type is **Alzheimer's Disease.** Most of the types of dementia are **progressive** and cannot be reversed.

There are **a few** types of dementia which **can be** stopped or reversed, and is one reason early diagnosis and intervention is important. Some causes of dementia that **can be reversed** by early intervention include brain tumors, low Vitamin B 12, blood imbalance of sugar, sodium, or calcium, and chronic alcohol abuse.

Besides problems with memory, **other symptoms** include deterioration in emotional behavior and skills required for calculation, abstract thinking, and judgment.

Stages of dementia include the following:

Early symptoms begin with forgetfulness. Some forgetfulness could be normal and does not progress. If it does continue to progress, there is a need for concern.

Next, is a period of **mild cognitive impairment** that involves forgetting recent events, impaired problem solving, difficulty performing more than one task at a time, and taking longer to perform a more complicated mental task. At this stage, the individual is **usually aware** of their forgetfulness. Not all people with mild cognitive impairment progress to dementia.

Next, the individual **forgets** the names of **familiar** objects, misplaces items, gets lost easily, starts to lose social skills, loses interest in activities previously enjoyed, and has difficulty performing mental activities, such as balancing a checkbook.

Then, the individual **forgets personal** events and self-identity, has changes in sleep patterns, poor judgment, and difficulty in preparing meals or driving. At this stage there, **also, may** be delusions, depression, or agitation.

In the **final stage**, the individual is unable to understand communications, recognize family members, or perform basic activities of daily living.

Diagnosis is made based upon the individual's history, present symptoms, and the results of a mental status examination. Since dementia is more common in individuals over 65, a thorough health care provider will **administer a mental status examine** from time to time. The test is easy to administer and does not mean that the healthcare provider suspects the patient may have dementia.

When dementia is suspected, **additional procedures** will be performed to rule out other causes of the symptoms. **Some of those other causes** include vitamin deficiencies, thyroid disease, brain tumor, HIV/AIDS, intoxication, depression, or anemia.

Treatment aims to control the symptoms of dementia, depending upon the underlying cause. Some **medications,** such as mood stabilizers, may be needed to help control behavioral problems. There are some **drugs,** such as Aricept or Namenda, that may be used to slow the worsening of symptoms.

As the condition progresses, keeping the individuals safe and making sure their basic needs are met are the primary goals. Some people with dementia tend to be restless and may wander, including during the nighttime (called **Sundown Syndrome**).

The **Alzheimer's Association (www.alz.org)** provides helpful suggestions on how to protect the individuals without restraining them. There are, also, **care units** that specialize in the care of individuals with dementia, when it becomes too difficult to care for them at home. Additionally, there are **respite services** available to assist families who are caring for someone with dementia at home.

So far, there are no concrete methods known to prevent dementia, except for some of the known causes that are treatable. Remaining **healthy and active,** both physically and mentally, is suggested to help delay the onset of symptoms.

REMINDERS:
Orientation:

- **Orientation based stimulation** is helpful, such as clocks, familiar objects, and calendars that highlight the current day.
- **Remind** individual of time, place, and person.
- **When communicating** talk slowly, clearly, and **repeat** important information.
- Provide **small pieces** of information, at a time.
- **Make sure** the information is understood.
- **Clarify** any misunderstood information.
- **Encourage reminiscence**. Photo albums are a handy tool.
- Try to maintain a **calm, quiet environment.**
- **Limit stimulation** by reducing noise and excessive lighting.
- **Allow time** for the individual to accomplish tasks.
- **Set up a regular schedule** for personal care, meals, and events.
- **Approach slowly** and in a calm manner, so as not to startle and upset the individual.

Safety:

- **Provide a safe environment** with clear pathways, handrails, and secure dangerous items, such as matches and knives.

- **Store medications** in a safe, locked cabinet.
- Think in terms of a **childproof** environment.
- **Provide an alarm system** to signal, if the individual wanders outdoors or to an unsafe area.
- **Orient** them to anything new in the environment.
- Use **out-of-reach locks** on doors.
- Low heeled, nonskid shoes provide safe **footwear.**
- **Provide a safe bathroom** environment with grab bars and shower bench.
- **Provide night lights** in bathroom, bedroom, and halls.
- **Provide supervision,** as needed, when bathing, preparing meals, and walking.
- Have individual wear an **ID bracelet** at all times.
- **Plan** what to do if individual becomes lost.
- Allow for **naps, but avoid** letting them sleep for an extended period of time during the day and end up not sleeping at night.
- Keep them occupied with some **planned activities** during the day.

Resources:

- The **Alzheimer's Association (www.alz.org)** provides support services and useful, practical information.

- **Support** the caregiver(s).
- **Involve** all willing family members and/ or friends in planning and caring for the individual, so the main caregiver does not become overwhelmed.
- **Utilize respite care services** such as adult daycare or paid help.
- Family and caregivers need to still **meet their own health and emotional needs.**
- **Utilize counseling** services and **support** groups.
- Do not be afraid to **consider long-term placement** as the dementia progresses or if the family/caregiver resources become exhausted.

CANCER:

Cancer is an uncontrolled growth of abnormal (malignant) body cells and can spread (metastasize) to other locations via the lymph system or the blood stream. It can be found in almost any body organ or tissue including the lungs, stomach, intestines, reproductive organs, skin, bones, blood, lymph nodes, and nerve tissue.

There are **many known causes,** such as chemicals, environmental toxins, excessive sunlight, obesity, radiation, infections, sexually transmitted diseases, and genetics. Because there are different types of cancer that are prevalent in different countries, diet seems to play a role in some cancers.

Symptoms vary according to its location. It may start as a **painless lump** if located in a superficial (near surface) area. Since **early signs** do not always include pain, some cancers can start to spread before they are discovered.

Some **other early signs** of cancer can be a cough, shortness of breath, chest pain, diarrhea, constipation, and/or blood in stool or urine. **Blood** should always be investigated. As you can see, these are very common symptoms that could indicate many different conditions, other than cancer. Some **other common symptoms** of cancer include fatigue, fever, loss of appetite, and weight loss. An indication that may imply cancer, is not just if these symptoms are present, but if they persist.

Not all cancers can be **prevented,** but it does help to eat a balanced diet, exercise, control weight, avoid tobacco, avoid heavy alcohol use, and control sun exposure. In other words, moderation is the key.

Since many cancers cannot be prevented, **early detection** can be a life saver. **Regular** medical examinations and cancer screenings, such as mammography and colonoscopy, help with early detection.

It can be scary to discover a sign of cancer, and it is a normal inclination for us to try to deny there may be a problem. However, **the sooner medical attention is sought the better.** If it isn't cancer, you will be preventing unnecessary worry. If it is cancer, the chances of achieving a cure or control with early treatment are better than if you wait.

Diagnosis is made by the use of blood tests, x-rays, CT and MRI scans, and biopsies. A **definitive diagnosis** can only be made with a biopsy. Scans help to find the exact location and size of the tumor(s).

I remember when I was pregnant with my first child, the doctor discovered a tumor attached to my uterus. He told me there was an 80% chance that the tumor was malignant. I didn't hear much of what he said after that statement. If you are undergoing tests and could possibly receive "bad news" from the doctor, it is best to **take someone with you for your appointment.** Then, if you have trouble hearing the news, your family member or friend can help ask questions and even take notes for you.

Treatment consists of **removal** of the cancer, if it is confined in a specific area that can be reached. Even if the cancer seems to be in a confined area, the surgeon will try to remove some healthy tissue around the tumor to avoid leaving any cancer cells.

Some of these surgeries, even if lifesaving, **may still cause some deformities.** There are **therapies and devices** to help the patient adapt.

Other therapies that may be used with or instead of surgery are radiation, chemotherapy, and certain medications. Sometimes the number of options from which a person needs to choose can be overwhelming. The individual, fortunate enough to have **supportive family members or friends,** should take advantage of their help to make decisions. The **American Cancer Society (www.cancer.org)**

and other cancer groups provide support services to help with decisions.

Radiation therapy is painless. Radiation equipment and techniques have improved over the years to limit collateral damage. However, the **skin** in the treated area may temporarily become sensitive and irritated. It helps to allow for plenty of rest and a well balanced diet.

Chemotherapy has come a long way over the past decades. More than 50 years ago, there were a few anti-cancerous drugs being used, essentially on an experimental basis. Patients who agreed to chemotherapy, at that time, were heroes. Most of them were not expected to live, however, they were willing to try this as a "last ditch effort". If it were not for these willing patients, doctors would not have been able to learn which medications, combinations of medications, and their doses would be most effective.

These drugs still have **side effects,** although doctors have learned how to control and minimize them. Health care professionals who work with chemotherapy patients have, also, learned how to help these patients deal with the side effects.

One side effect of chemotherapy is its effects on the **immune system**. Chemotherapy causes a weakening of the immune system, making patients more vulnerable when fighting **infections**. People receiving chemotherapy need to avoid anyone with colds and flu.

There are some medications that have been discovered which **reduce the risk** of certain types of cancer and their recurrence. Some of these medications have been used to reduce the risk of cancer of the breast, prostate, or colon. Your healthcare provider can give you further information about these medications.

There are some **alternative treatments** that have not been proven to be effective against cancer. Some may be harmless, but they may delay the use of an effective treatment or cause patients to waste their money on treatments that have no benefits. Always discuss the use of alternative therapies with your medical provider, before choosing them.

Palliative care is a multidiscipline approach to control physical, emotional, psychosocial, and spiritual symptoms. Palliative care should not be confused with hospice care. One does not have to be dying to utilize these services.

REMINDERS:

- Do not hesitate to **ask questions** of healthcare personnel. You will progress better if you are well informed and know what to expect.
- Do not hesitate to **share feelings.** Just having someone you trust listen to your concerns can be helpful.
- Take advantage of **support groups** and/or **counseling,** as needed.

- Utilize **American Cancer Society (www.cancer. org)** for information and services available in your community. Reach to Recovery (breast cancer) and Man to Man (prostate cancer) are two programs offered by the cancer society.
- In addition to therapies and medications, relaxation exercises, music therapy, and other **diversions to reduce anxiety and pain** can be helpful.
- **Keep appointments** for follow-up care, laboratory tests, and other treatments.
- **Hospice** not only provides medical and nursing services for terminally ill patients, but it also provides legal and spiritual counseling.
- Maintain a **nutritional diet.**
- **Notify primary medical provider** if experiencing nausea, vomiting, or diarrhea.
- Use anti-nausea and/or diarrhea medication, as needed.
- **Use supplemental** high protein, high caloric feedings to maintain nutrition.
- **Follow special dietary requirements,** as advised by your medical provider.
- **Avoid hot, spicy foods**, as instructed.
- Eat **smaller, more frequent meals** in a relaxed, quiet environment to help your appetite.
- **Mouth care** before meals improves the appetite.

- **Report any blood** in stools or urine to your medical provider.
- Avoid the use of **stiff toothbrushes.**
- Apply **petroleum jelly or cocoa butter** to lips.
- **If blood count is abnormal**, avoid eating raw vegetables. Do not share utensils.
- **Cool** drinks, popsicles, and ice cream help soothe the mouth.
- **Notify** your medical provider if **any sores** develop in your mouth.
- **Cleanse skin** with mild soap, warm water, and pat skin dry with a towel.
- **Follow directions** for skin care of any irradiated areas.
- **Avoid rubbing and scratching** the skin and avoid **adhesive** tape and **sun** exposure.
- Use soft, loose fitting **clothing** for comfort.
- Report any **skin breakdown** to your medical provider.
- Avoid contact with others who have **infections.**
- **ALWAYS WASH YOUR HANDS**.
- Caregivers should always wash their hands.
- Use an **electric razor** rather than a safety razor to avoid cuts.
- **Wash hair** with mild shampoo and avoid use of curlers, dryers, harsh brushing and hair spray.

- **If hair is lost**, it will grow back. **Use of** a wig and/or scarves will help you adjust to the hair loss.
- The **American Cancer Society (www.cancer. org)** web site offers wigs, scarves, bras and breast forms to choose from, for purchase..
- Scarves and loose clothing can be used to cover **surgical area scars or protheses**.
- Some hospice agencies have supplies, such as dressings and wigs, as well as equipment, such as walkers available for rent or for a small fee.

CHAPTER XI

MEDICATION THERAPY

As we grow older, most of us have an increasing need to take medications on a regular basis. The more medications you are taking, the more careful you need to be when handling them.

There are **five rights** to keep in mind.

- Right Person
- Right Medication
- Right Dose
- Right Time
- Right Route

Usually the **right person** should not be an issue. However, there are some patients who take medicine that was prescribed for a friend or relative. The other person tells them that they had the same problem and this medication "really helped". I can't express just how **dangerous** this practice can be. Health professionals not only prescribe a particular medication for a particular disease or symptom, but they also consider the patient's age, size, and medical history, just to mention a few factors.

All prescribed medications should be **kept in their original container,** so there is a way to identify the **right medication**.

I am sure you have noticed that there are many pills that look alike and are easily confused. Some people have the habit of placing all of their pills together in a baggy. That is a good way to get pills mixed up and end up taking the wrong medication. Also be aware which meds need to be taken before meals and which need to be taken with food. There are cost effective **medicine boxes** that can be used to help you remember to take your medications at the **right times**, under the right circumstances.

When I worked as a home care nurse, we would have patients bring out all the drugs they were taking, when we admitted them to our services. It was not uncommon for them to bring out a 12 square inch storage box filled with medications and herbs. Frequently, we would find the individual was taking two to three **duplicate meds,** of which their primary physician was unaware because different physicians had ordered them.

Duplication of medications can be a common occurrence, since all of us see more than one physician. Some seniors can be taking duplicate drugs and not realize it, nor realize the dangers involved.

Make sure you understand the **information** about all of the drugs you are taking, including herbal medications. Also, pay attention to warnings of **interactions** between medications, foods, and herbs. You could be causing overdoses or interfering with the desired drug action.

We need to make sure **all** our doctors have a current list of **all** our medications. The wisest thing is to carry a **current**

medication list with us, which comes in handy not only for scheduled medical visits, but also if we have to go to an ER or urgent care.

Read all directions about when and how to take each medication. Make sure that each medication is taken in the **right amount** and at the **right time.**

REMINDER: Medication boxes help you remember to take each med correctly and not take a double dose.

The main **routes** that most people are going to use with self administration of medications are **orally** (by mouth) or **topically** (ointment, cream or trans dermal patch). Another route that some people have to learn to use is **injections**. For example, diabetics who need to take insulin learn to administer their own injections.

When taking a **newly prescribed** medication, **read all the instructions** you receive from the doctor and pharmacist. Pay attention to suggested times to take, any foods or other medications that may interfere with its actions, any precautions, or any contraindications.

Avoid missing a dose, but if you should miss one, **do not take a double dose** with the next administration. The pharmacy instructions will usually tell you what to do if a dose is missed, however, do not hesitate to **ask questions** of your health professional or pharmacist.

Many people forget to consider **herbal medications,** but some of them may contain the same ingredients as prescription medications and/or can enhance or inhibit drug actions. If you don't understand something, ask your physician or pharmacist.

Pharmacists are a great resource for drug information. Don't forget to read the handouts you receive when you renew a prescription. That has a lot of useful information, including how and when to take the medication.

If you are having **trouble swallowing pills**, ask if you can take the medication in a different form, that would be easier to take. Many drugs are available in more than one form. **Do not** take it on yourself to **crush a tablet or open a capsule** because there are some medications whose action could be altered if the tablet or capsule is changed, especially if it is a long-acting medication.

If you are taking **several different medications**, it would be helpful to **keep a chart** for which meds you are to take at which time during the day. It would be helpful to **carry a copy** of that chart with you in case you ever need to go to the hospital or for when you make a doctor's visit.

Wash your hands before preparing your medications. If you are preparing meds for someone else, you definitely need to wash your.

When taking a liquid preparation or preparing an injection, measure carefully. It helps to hold the container at **eye level** so you can see accurately. Pour liquids out of a bottle with the **label facing outward,** so the label does not become stained.

Do not use meds beyond their **expiration date.** Do not discard meds in the toilet or garbage due to environmental and drug abuse concerns. Most communities have arranged for **periodic collection** of medications. Your local pharmacist will probably be able to inform you about times and locations of such collections.

If you are giving yourself **injections**, take extra care when disposing of the syringes and needles. **NEVER** leave them lying around where you or someone else can get a needle stick. To avoid a finger stick, **do not** try to **recap** the needle.

Dispose of needles in a **puncture proof container**. Use a hard plastic bottle such as a laundry soap bottle, but not a soft plastic bottle that contained milk or orange juice. (Needles can penetrate the soft plastic.) **Seal** the container before disposal. Some communities have a special place to dispose of syringes. Your local pharmacist should be able to inform you of local regulations. **Do not reuse** needles or syringes.

Transdermal (via skin) patches have become a popular route for administration of certain drugs. The **skin area** needs to be cleaned before application of the patch. Always **remove any older** patches before applying a new one. **Do not cut** a patch in half because that may affect the dose delivery rate or even dry out the medicine base so it cannot be absorbed.

Take all doses of **antibiotics,** as ordered. If all doses are not taken, the organism may be weakened, but not killed and could come back stronger. **Do not take** any antibiotics that are **not prescribed** for you. There are some US citizens who purchase antibiotics in Mexico and take them for conditions caused by viruses, such as a cold, that do not respond to antibiotics. Such practices contribute to the creation of **"super bugs".** Super bugs lead to the antibiotic resistant conditions we are observing today.

If you notice any **unexpected reaction** to the medication, such as a rash, **report it immediately** to your medical professional. That, also, is true if the medication does not provide the expected results after taking a few doses.

REMINDERS:

- **Follow instructions** regarding use of medications with alcohol, tobacco, caffeine, or herbs.
- Note **expiration** dates.
- **Store** in cool, dry cabinet, out of reach of children.
- **Refrigerate** if medication is to be kept at a lower temperature.
- **Discard** all expired medications.
- **Check medication** bottle for name, dose, and time before taking.
- **Follow special instructions,** such as before or after meals, or with or without food.
- Use measuring spoon or calibrated cup for **accuracy** of measuring liquid meds.

- Use a **pill crusher,** if needed, and mix with water, juice, or soft food, if so indicated by physician or pharmacist.
- Use **medication boxes** to help remember to take your meds at the proper times, and do not miss a dose or take a medication twice.
- **Avoid removing** your meds from their prescription bottles and mixing them together in one container or bag.
- Remember the **five rights** of medication administration: (person, medication, dose, time, and route).

CHAPTER XII

HOSPITALS/MEDICAL CENTERS

Hospitals/ Medical Centers provide a variety of services for both inpatient and outpatient care. These services are provided by specialized staff. Most hospitals are **nonprofit,** but some are **for profit** facilities.

There are many different **types of hospitals**. The various types include community, county, or district medical centers. Others are run by a private group, such as a religious organization, others by an insurance group or a health organization. Some of these hospitals offer a broad range of medical services, and others are specialty hospitals.

Some communities, with several hospitals, will designate certain ones to provide a **specialty center** in order to control medical costs and avoid duplication of services. Some of those centers include cardiac, orthopedic, or burn care. This system helps contain costs because the specialty equipment can be located in just one center, and the staff develops an expertise in that particular area. There are other hospitals that specialize in just one area, such as psychiatric, children, or geriatrics.

Most community medical centers provide a wide diversity of services. **Outpatient services** usually include emergency, minor surgery, and other treatments that do not require hospitalization. **Inpatient services** usually include medical-surgical nursing, intensive care, cardiac care, surgery, pediatrics, labor and delivery, rehabilitation, and radiology. Departments that provide **support services** include laboratory, pharmacy, and dietary.

Many medical centers are linked to **medical and/or nursing schools,** and provide clinical experience for the students. Most of these facilities recognize there is a mutual benefit providing learning experiences for students. Not only do the students gain valuable experience, but their questions help keep the nursing and medical staff up to date. When you have another pair of eyes watching you and your technique, you are motivated to provide the highest quality of care.

Organizational structure:

Most medical centers are **organized** into several departments headed by an administration. Over the years, the titles of the administrators and managers have changed, but the responsibilities tend to remain the same. The **CEO (chief executive officer)** usually has a minimum of a masters degree in hospital administration.

One, who watches TV medical programs, would get the impression that it is the physician who runs the hospital and supervises the nursing staff, but there is nothing farther from the truth. Most medical centers have a process where by the **physician applies** for medical staff membership and privileges. Some physicians will have staff membership at more than one hospital. Each hospital has certain rules and regulations that must be followed in order to maintain staff membership. Some of the regulations are set by the hospital's medical staff, while other regulations are required of all the staff, by the hospital. The administrator of the medical staff is the **chief of staff,** which may be a permanent, salaried position by the hospital or a temporary, unpaid position. The unpaid type of position is usually an elected position by the medical staff.

Some hospitals, such as County or HMOs, have salaried medical staff. In recent years, some hospitals have been hiring paid medical staff to supplement the medical staff with privileges. These staff members are called **hospitalists** who, with the approval of the patient's physician, provide medical care while the patient is hospitalized. They also care for patients who do not have their own physician. Hospitalists do not provide care for patients once they have been discharged. Advantages of a hospitalist staff are closer patient supervision, better coordination of medical care, and more office time for the primary care physicians. Besides the use of hospitalists, many hospitals contract with a group of physicians to provide medical services for some specialty areas, such as the emergency department.

Working with the CEO are several **vice presidents (VP).** The number and responsibilities of the vice presidents varies depending upon the size and needs of the particular institution. The VPs, along with the CEO, are responsible to insure that their hospital areas are operating in compliance with all government rules and regulations, of which there are many.

There is always a **VP of Finance,** who is responsible for all of the financial aspects of the institution.

Usually, all of the patient care departments are administered by someone with a nursing background **(VP of Patient Care Services),** who usually has a minimum of a masters in nursing and extensive clinical experience. Pharmacy, rehabilitation, dietary, and human resources may report to the patient care VP or be grouped together with another VP, depending upon the size of the medical center.

There may also be another division for **support services** that might include plant and maintenance, housekeeping, computer services, patient records, imaging/radiology, and laboratory services. A fast growing hospital department is informatics, which combines health, computer, and information sciences to acquire, store, retrieve, and use information to meet the needs of patients.

Besides an administrator, these departments will usually have a **director/manager** to head them. Laboratory and Imaging will each have a **contracted physician** with a specialty in that particular discipline. The physician, as head of the department, will usually share the management of the department with a technician, who also specializes in the same discipline.

The **Division of Patient Care** comprises the major part of a medical center. (Actually a hospital/ medical center would be like a giant outpatient clinic without the nursing staff, because there would be no one to care for the patients.) The nursing departments are directed by nurse managers. Today, most hospitals operate on 12 hour shifts for the inpatient departments. The staff is usually composed of registered nurses and certified nursing assistants. Each department has an RN who is in charge of the unit for the entire shift.

From time to time, hospitals will try to reduce the RN staff and replace them with a less prepared staff, in an effort to reduce expenses. Over the years, studies have shown that a larger RN staff provides better patient safety, as well as better patient outcomes.

Patient care **support units** are managed by someone with expertise in the discipline that is providing the service, for example a dietitian, pharmacist, therapist, or computer technologist.

As previously stated, many people are under the impression that the doctor runs the hospital and supervises the hospital personnel. Actually, the physician **works with** the hospital personnel to provide patient care.

When physicians admit patients to the hospital, they agree to **follow the policies and procedures,** approved by the hospital administration and the medical staff executive committee. These policies and procedures are based on current medical/nursing research and regulations, required by various federal and state agencies that impact health care. If a hospital is accredited, it will also have addition regulations that must be maintained. To meet all of these regulations, medical centers are expected to set up and maintain **protocols,** that are expected to be **practiced by all of the hospital and medical staff**.

The physician **submits admission orders** for the patient. The physician then either turns over medical care for the patient to the hospital medical staff, such as the hospitalists, or will continue to provide the medical care. Each hospital will have its own protocols on the role of the hospitalist.

The **nursing staff** not only implements the medical orders, but also develops and initiates an **individualized nursing care plan** for the patient. The nursing care plan includes both physician and nursing orders, which are personalized to meet the needs of the individual patient. The care plan takes into consideration not only the patient's medical and physical needs, but also their psychosocial needs.

Registered nurses are highly **skilled practitioners.** They provide many of the procedures that are ordered for the patient, i.e., catheterizations, intramuscular and intravenous injections, wound care, and the provision of comfort and pain relief. They are the ones who usually perform these skills in the hospital setting.

A major responsibility for the nurse is to **document** the implementation of the care plan, patient observations, and patient outcomes that result from the care. In addition to performing procedures, the **RN functions** as a teacher, coordinator, manager, and patient advocate.

The nurses are the ones who **monitor the patient's condition, 24/7,** and notify the appropriate physician when medical attention is required. The nurse, also, assigns and supervises the nursing assistants when providing patient care. The nursing assistants usually perform basic care such as bathing, feeding, and taking vital signs (blood pressure, pulse, and temperatures).

The **RN is responsible** for making sure that all lab and X-ray procedures are ordered, that all medications have arrived from the pharmacy, and are administered as ordered. The nurse, also, **observes** the patient for any side effects from medications and treatments. The nurse **coordinates** the nursing care to be sure that it is delivered at the appropriate times, and the patient receives treatments and procedures, as ordered, from other hospital departments. Nursing works to **coordinate all care** so everything gets done, and the patient still has some time to rest and recuperate.

Most medical centers have **transport services** to transfer patients to other departments when they are scheduled for procedures, such as X-rays. Frequently, therapists will come to the patient's room to provide therapy, unless special equipment is needed. If the patient is scheduled for surgery, the surgery department will usually transport the patient to and from the area.

The nursing staff provides a great deal of **education** for patients and their families. They want to make sure that the patients understand the important precautions about their medications and how to perform new procedures and/ or exercises when discharged.

If there is any **follow-up care** needed after discharge, the nurses will make suggestions to the doctor that home care or outpatient services may be helpful. One problem with the **shortening of hospital stays** is that patients can be sent home before they have enough time to learn to care for themselves. We then end up seeing those same patients being readmitted because they didn't understand how to care for their wound, or take certain precautions to prevent a relapse. There are some complicated conditions, like Diabetes, that require the patient to return for additional classes before they are able to independently manage their care.

Frequently the nurse needs to **advocate** for the patient and even sometimes for their family members. Sometimes, the nurse needs to be the bad guy and shoo out visitors so the patient can get some rest, especially if one or more visitor(s) are argumentative.

There are, also, times when the patient did not understand what the doctor was telling them, but they were hesitant to ask questions. Most nurses will try to be available when doctors are making rounds, so they will be aware of what the doctor says. Then they can clarify for the patients what the doctor was telling them

If the doctor has given some **bad news,** the nurse can be especially helpful. Sometimes, patients and their families have a hard time getting their minds around the bad news, especially if they were not expecting a problem.

Nurses **record** any questions the patients may have, so the doctors are aware that they need to spend extra time explaining the information. If there is a serious concern, the nurse frequently will phone the physician to be sure the physician understands the concern. These are just two examples of when nurses are needed to advocate for the patient.

One of the main areas where **nurses act as advocates** is making sure that everyone providing patient care is **following protocols,** such as hand-washing and other safety measures. This includes the medical staff. Many hospital protocols are developed to provide safety for patients. Most of these are set up as a series of checks, so if there is a break in protocol at one point, it can be rectified to prevent harm.

Medication administration is an example:

- The **doctor inputs orders** for medications into the computer system. (There may still be some small healthcare facilities where the doctor needs to hand write the orders.)
- The **nurse then acknowledges** the order and makes sure the dosage is appropriate for the particular patient.
- If there is a **discrepancy**, the nurse needs to contact the physician about the order and/or consult with the pharmacist.
- The medication order is automatically **transmitted to the pharmacy** when the doctor inputs it into the computer.
- The **pharmacist is also responsible** to make sure that the order is appropriate for the patient

and is compatible with the patient's other medications.

- When dispensing the medication, the **pharmacist verifies** that the order contains the correct medication, dosage, route, and time.
- When preparing the prescription, protocol requires the pharmacist to **check the medication at least 3 times** to be sure there is no mistake.
- Most medical centers use **computerized systems** to verify that the correct patient is receiving the correct medication at the right time.
- When the medication is administered, the **nurse will first verify** this information.
- (If a hospital does not have a computerized system for medication administration, the **nurse is responsible** to make sure the patient, drug, dosage, time, and route are all correct.)

When everyone follows the protocols, errors are kept at a minimum. If an error does occur, it is usually a minor one. (I have observed that when a serious error occurs, there was usually more than one person who "dropped the ball".)

What To Expect If You Or A Family Member Is Admitted To The Hospital.

How well prepared you are for a hospitalization is going to depend upon the reason for the hospitalization, i.e., a planned surgery versus an unexpected emergency. **Take**

advantage of any **informational sessions** that may be offered to you before admission. Planned surgeries usually have pre-admission sessions that provide important information to help you prepare for your hospital stay. Hopefully, you are also provided written information to reinforce the session. Nurses have found that the better prepared someone is before surgery, the more rapidly they recover.

Doctors are frequently given **handouts** from the hospitals. It might be helpful to ask if there is a handout available. **Written information** is especially helpful because you have it available to refer back to later. If there are no written instructions, you might find it helpful to write some notes to help remember details.

A **planned hospitalization,** frequently, includes registering the patient beforehand. If that has not been done, the patient will have to go to the **admissions department** when they arrive to be admitted. The exception would be, if they are admitted through the emergency department. No matter when the **formal admission** occurs, it is helpful to have information about **insurances and/or Medicare and Medicaid.** Don't forget to bring your **list of medications,** including over-the-counter and herbal medications. Do not assume the doctor is going to remember all your current medications. This way the nurse is alerted and can remind the doctor to order your routine medications.

If there is a **living will and/or medical power of attorney,** the hospital will need a copy, so bring it with you. It is difficult to implement a living will without knowing the patient's exact wishes. We have many people from out of town who tell us that their living will is securely locked in a safe at home. Frequently, people are so protective of the document, it is not available when needed.

The admission process to the **patient room** is going to vary according to the individual hospital or medical center. Basically, you will be escorted to the room and oriented to the location of items and shown how to work equipment, such as the call light, TV, and bed. If the hospital utilizes a transport service, the transporter will probably not stay with you, but will make sure you are safely situated, and then notify the nurse that you have arrived.

The nurse or aide will come to help you, within a few minutes after your arrival. Everyone who comes in contact with you should introduce themselves and let you know their role in your treatment. Do not hesitate to have them repeat something or ask for clarification.

The hospital staff are used to using medical jargon and sometimes forget you may not be familiar with the words. The **RNs**, responsible for your care, need to be clear about their role since they are the ones who you should be talking to, **if there is a problem**. You are entitled to know everyone who will be giving you your medications and/or treatments.

That **does not mean you cannot ask** anyone else about when you should be getting certain services or letting them know you need help, such as pain medication. **Everyone works together** and, even if they are not responsible for a certain task, they will know who to ask to get what you need. Many hospitals have a **white board** in patients' rooms, which will have the name of the RN and aide for that particular room and any other vital information for patient and family reference.

The **aide will assist** the patient with undressing and getting comfortable. The aide also records a checklist of the belongings, the patient is going to keep at the hospital If your family brings in any other items, it is wise to ask the nurse to record it.

The **aide will, also, check** vital signs and any other procedure that is needed for the patient. The aide is responsible for **orienting** the patient to the room and equipment, teaching how to operate the bed, call system, TV, and bathroom. The aide will then notify the nurse that the patient has arrived, and get water for the patient and anything else that he/she may need or want.

The nurse will try to see the new patient, as soon as possible. Medical orders and admission information is, usually, already available. Those **orders need to be acknowledged** by the RN before they are initiated. Currently, many hospitals have changed from a paper record to an electronic record for the patient.

The RN will perform a **head to toe assessment,** with a focus on the patient's medical diagnosis. For example, if the patient has pneumonia, the nurse will spend extra time listening to the patient's lung sounds, and checking for other signs that may indicate some other complications of pneumonia. This initial assessment helps to **provide a baseline** for the nurses and physicians, to use to evaluate the patient's status from time to time. During the assessment, the nurse will assess the patient for **pain, risk for falls, skin breakdown,** and **injury**. The RN, also, obtains information about the diet at home and bowel, hygiene, and sleep habits.

The **initial nursing assessment, also, includes social information,** such as family and significant others, contact information, and predominant language. Also included, are the patient's mental alertness, usual activity levels, any ambulatory needs, and spiritual needs. In addition, any assistive devices needed, such as hearing aides and glasses. The patient's use of alcohol, cigarettes, and/or drugs are noted.

All of this data is **documented** and used to provide a basis for the formulation of the individualized nursing care plan. The care plan helps **provide consistency,** no matter which nurse is providing care, throughout the patient's hospitalization.

Besides the specific physical needs of the patient, the care plan will include **teaching needs**. Based on this initial assessment and medical orders, the **RN makes referrals,** as appropriate, to therapy (PT, OT, SLP), radiology/imaging, laboratory, dietary, and pharmacy. The nurse will also **remind the physician** to order medications and/or diet that is consistent with what the patient is accustomed to at home.

Discharge planning for the patient begins shortly after admission. Social services work with the medical and nursing staff to plan for when the patient will be discharged to home or to another care facility, assistive living, or rehabilitation. **Home care** is always an option for someone who prefers going home. The patient and/or family should be involved early in this process and so they are well prepared before the patient is discharged.

Today, most hospitals operate on **12-hour shifts** (7-7). The oncoming nurse meets with the off-going nurse to review the patients they are sharing, to promote consistency of care. The staff works to make the transition of care as smooth as possible.

Hospitals promote a **consistent communication system** to facilitate accuracy and completeness of vital information. This system is especially critical at the change of shifts, when a patient is transferred from one nursing unit to another, or transferred from one department to another, i.e., patient room to x-ray or surgery.

Daily routine for the nursing assistant, usually, includes routine vital signs (pulse, temperature, respiration, blood pressure), blood sugars, baths, meal setup, and bedtime care. They, also, assist patients with ambulating (walking), changing positions in bed, and moving to the chair and to the bathroom.

Meals are usually brought to patients' rooms by the **dietary staff**. Since they have not been trained to assist patients, they will just deliver the meal trays to the room. The **nursing assistant** follows closely behind to help the patients sit up so they can eat. **If someone does not appear** shortly after the tray arrives, use the call light to summon assistance.

Sometimes, the aide gets tied up in another patient's room. All of the staff on a nursing unit **work together,** so if one nurse or aide gets busy with another patient, others will step in to help. The staff coordinate their meal breaks so the other staff can watch their patients while they are gone. The staff nurses, each **carry zone phones,** so they can be contacted easily.

The **daily routine of the staff RN** includes:

- Receive **report** on assigned patients.
- Review **patient records**.
- **Plan schedule** for the shift.
- Perform head to toe **assessments** on all assigned patients.
- Obtain vital signs and blood sugar **results**.
- Make sure all **equipment** is working properly, including IVs.
- Administer **medications** at appropriate times.
- **Contact** physicians, as needed.
- Verify that patients receive **scheduled tests and treatments.**
- Perform **nursing treatments** at appropriate times.
- Arrange implementation of any **new doctors' orders.**
- **Supervise aides** provision of patient care.
- Make sure **safety precautions** are always maintained.
- **Monitor** patients on a routine basis.

- Check each patient **at least every hour**, even during the night.
- **(Intensive care units** maintain a more constant observation of the patients.)
- **Contact physician,** if patient shows signs of deterioration.
- Implement **emergency measures,** when needed.
- **Document** all nursing care.

If you have questions or feel you are not receiving proper care, **the RN** is an **excellent resource.** Some times the patient waits for their doctor to come to see them, when the nurse could have solved the problem much sooner. Frequently, the doctor has to seek out the nurse, anyway, to take care of the issue. If it is a problem that involves the physician, the nurse will let you know, and if it is something that can't wait, will contact the physician for you. Sometimes, the nurse can obtain an order from the physician and implement it much sooner, than if you waited for the physician to come in to see you.

CHAPTER XIII

HOME HEALTH CARE

Home Health Care has been available, in different forms, almost since the beginning of time. Its use has increased in the last few decades, as a result of efforts toward managing health care costs. With **earlier discharges from the hospital**, patients are sent home with further **need for treatments, therapy, and information.** Some people need to go to a rehabilitation hospital or nursing home, until they are able to take care of themselves at home. Home health care **provides another option** for these people, especially those who have family members or friends who can assist them. It is recognized that most people **prefer to stay at home** to recuperate, or if they have a chronic illness. Patients usually **thrive better at home**.

There are **third party payers** who pay for home health care, depending upon the circumstances. They recognize that care at home is **more cost effective** and generally **safer,** than in a care facility. Some of the **third party payers** that do reimburse for care at home are Medicaid, Medicare, long-term care insurance, and a few private insurances.

When receiving home care services, be sure to notify the agency if you make a change in your primary payor, because the agency will need to gain approval from your current payor to provide services. This helps to prevent any interruption in services.

These agencies are very specific about what care will be covered by them and their rules for participation. Any care not covered, such as nurse aide care, could be provided if the patient chooses to pay for it.

Medicare provides a clear example of these rules, which is called **Conditions of Participation.** The basic Medicare criteria includes:

- Valid Medicare client.
- Certified agency provides the services.
- The services are reasonable and necessary.
- Under physician's signed orders.
- Patient is homebound.
- Plan of care includes skilled services.
- Services take place in patient's residence.

Reasonable and necessary services are based upon the patient's current medical, psychiatric, and/or surgical condition. It is expected that these **services** are **temporary and intermittent.** In other words, they will not go on forever and services will not be 24/7.

The **Plan of Care** is established and reviewed periodically by the physician. The physician's plan of care and documentation in the patient's record must verify that the services have been provided, but also, that they were appropriate for the patient's condition.

Homebound means that the patient is not able to to leave home **without considerable effort,** and that this status is due to the patient's **current** illness or injury. This does not mean that the patient needs to be completely disabled, but it does mean that the **patient needs assistance** from someone or with an appliance, such as a walker. It is considered acceptable that the patient **would be allowed** to keep any medical appointments or attend adult day care. It is, also, **accepted** that the individual can leave the home for short, infrequent periods for non medical reasons, such as for religious services.

Some examples of **reasons for homebound** status related to a current medical condition include:

- Impaired mobility
- Blindness
- Mental confusion
- Risk for infection
- Psychiatric problems

The professional caregivers are expected to document the homebound status of the patient, on a regular basis. If the patient progresses to the point where **staying home is no longer necessary,** the patient is discharged. Usually by that time, the services are no longer necessary, or services can be rendered in an outpatient facility.

There are **three factors** that help determine homebound status:

- Patient is essentially **confined to home.**
- Confinement is **related to** a medical or physical condition.
- Absences from home are **infrequent** or are for **medical treatment**.

The **patient's residence** is where the person happens to be living, at the time of treatment. So if the patient's daughter is caring for the parent at her home during the time of services, that is considered the patient's residence. However, if the patient is a resident in an assisted living facility or nursing home, that is already licensed to provide skilled services, they are not eligible for home health services.

Skilled Services are provided by licensed nurses and/or therapists. Some examples of **skilled nursing** are wound care, catheter care, intravenous therapy, observation, evaluation, and teaching about medical conditions and medications. Psychiatric nursing care by a certified psychiatric nurse is also reimbursable. **Therapy** services include evaluation, teaching, therapeutic exercises, treatments, management, and evaluation of the therapeutic program and a maintenance program. The therapy, also, includes helping patients adapt their environment to meet their needs and help them adapt to their environment. Additionally, **medical social services** are available to help patients access community resources that might be needed.

Each home care patient is assigned a **case manager** to coordinate the services being received. If there is a need for skilled nursing, the RN will be the case manager. If skilled nursing is not involved, one of the therapists may take on the role of case manager.

As long as there is a need for skilled services, **home health aide services** can be provided, if there is a documented need. The **aide** services include assistance with activities of daily living, such as bathing. The aides must be **supervised by** the RN or therapist, who is providing the skilled services in the home. If both nursing and therapy are providing services, the RN will supervise the aide.

Clients tend to **value the aide services** more that the skilled services, probably because the aide provides more direct and personal care. The case managers will remind clients, that when skilled services are no longer necessary, aide services will, also, be discontinued; so the patients are better prepared when it happens.

If there is **still a need or desire** for continued aide services, there are usually other agencies that can provide such services for a fee. And, of course, if the client has **Medicaid services,** they may still be able to qualify for personnel care services.

Some **additional services,** that may help seniors remain in their homes, are meal programs, respite care, adult day care, senior centers, housekeeping, shopping, and transportation services. There are agencies that provide many of these services for a fee.

Medicare will also reimburse for some **durable medical equipment.** Pharmacies and medical equipment stores are familiar with equipment that is reimbursable and can help with the application to obtain the reimbursement.

I recommend you **shop around** for the best prices for medical equipment, especially if you have to pay for it yourself. There can be a wide range of prices for medical equipment. There are also **community agencies** that might be able to help. The **social worker** is a good resource to check with, when starting your search.

This gives you an idea of the basic requirements of Medicare for home care reimbursement. **Private insurances,** including long-term insurance, each have their own requirements, that vary from the Medicare rules. Insurance companies require **written approval** be obtained by the home care agency before providing any services.

Medicaid home care services vary from state to state. Medicaid patients are usually assigned a **case manager** who frequently arranges for home care services. Medicaid agencies do recognize that home care is cost effective.

If the patient needs continuing care in the home, the Medicaid case manager will arrange for personal care that includes not only bathing, but, also, meals and sometimes housekeeping for Medicaid approved clients. If a Medicaid client is also **Medicare eligible** and **needs skilled services,** then Medicare takes over the reimbursement during that time.

If your doctor does order **skilled home health care** for you, be aware that the **initial visit** will be longer than any of the subsequent visits. One reason is because there are **several forms and procedures, required** by State and Federal governments, that need to be completed. Additionally, a more **comprehensive medical assessment** must be performed to develop an accurate plan of care for the patient.

You will be asked to have **all medications** (prescribed, over-the-counter, & herbs) available, so the home care case manager (RN or therapist) has a complete list for the physician and staff who will be providing care. This is a good time to ensure you do not have duplicate medications of which the physician is not aware.

Part of the initial visit is a **home safety assessment**. The nurse or therapist will make sure the home is safe for you, especially if there are any disabilities/weaknesses related to your illness or injury. Another goal of the safety assessment is to make sure the **home is safe** enough for the patient **to receive home care**. The **Safety Precautions section in Chapter VII** of this book discusses details on how to keep a safe home environment.

This visit is a good time to let the case manager know about any **advanced directives,** such as a medical power of attorney and a living will, that the patient may have. The case manager will ask you about **your wishes related to resuscitation**. The agency will, also, need a copy of each advanced directive document on file, so your wishes can be included in the plan of care. That way, everyone who comes to your home from the agency will be aware of your wishes. If you ever make any changes in these documents, be sure to **update the information** with the agency nurse or therapist.

On the initial visit, the case manager will provide you with a copy of the **Client Bill of Rights and Responsibilities**. The case manager will highlight some of the important rights for you and ask if you have any questions. However, the case manager will realize that your focus, at that time, will be more on the care that you need, and not on that form. It is recommend that you take some time later, when you are not feeling rushed, to reread the document more thoroughly. After reading it, **write down any questions** that you may think of to ask the nurse or therapist, during the **next visit**. As a matter of fact, write down **any questions** you may think about regarding any aspect of your care, so you do not forget to ask them.

Notice that the document is **titled Client's rights and responsibilities.** As with all rights, there are accompanying responsibilities. Patients always have the **right** to be given **information** about their condition and treatments, but they also have the **responsibility** to provide information about their condition, that can affect their recovery.

They have the right to be **respected** by the agency employees, but they also have the responsibility to be respectful of the staff. They have a responsibility to maintain a **safe environment,** not only for themselves, but also for the agency staff, who are making the visits.

Before leaving the first visit, the nurse or therapist will **initiate the treatment or therapy,** that has been ordered by the physician. The case manager will, also, begin teaching you and your caregiver about your therapy so that, as you recover, you can take responsibility for your own care.

At the end of the initial visit, the case manager will usually leave a **folder** at your home, containing copies of forms you have signed, including a service agreement between you and the agency. Additionally, there may be some other forms, such as a list of your medications, your plan of care, and a plan for the home health aide. **Do not throw** this folder away or misplace it because it is there, not only, for your information, but also, to be used by the agency staff .

The **follow up visits** will be much shorter than the initial one. The plan of care will determine the length of each visit; usually between 30 to 60 minutes.

Depending upon the intensity of your therapy, the **visit frequency** may be anywhere from as much as 4-5 times a week to as little as once a week. As you progress, the visits become less frequent.

Most agencies will try to **schedule** these **visits** ahead of time, so you don't have any conflicting appointments. Home care personnel will usually give you an approximate arrival time because they cannot always predict any delays at another patient's home or in traffic. Usually they aim to arrive within 15-30 minutes of the scheduled time. If the delay is going to be longer, either the staff member or the office will try to contact you, so you know when to expect the visit.

One thing that surprises home care patients, is most home care staff are **available 24 hours a day 7 days a week.** Some treatments, such as wound care or intravenous antibiotic therapy, require visits twice a day at the beginning. There are also times when the patient runs into a problem and needs an extra visit.

Also, some patients need to be seen immediately after they have been discharged from the healthcare facility. Depending on the size of the home care agency, it will have one or two **nurses on call** to handle these situations. Most nurses don't mind going out on these calls because the patients and their families are usually so appreciative.

During my years as a home care nurse, I was **impressed at how well** clients and their caregivers were able to manage their care at home, including the higher tech types of treatments. They tend to be **more conscientious** when a treatment involves their own body or that of their loved one. Not only is receiving care at home more **cost effective,** it tends to be **safer,** because the clients are in their own familiar surroundings, where they get better rest, and are in an environment of lower risk for infections.

If the senior is cared for at home, be aware that the **main caregiver(s)** needs a lot of support. Depending upon how ill the senior is, the care giver **may need some relief.** Frequently, they may not get a full night's sleep. The lack of sleep can accumulate to where the caregiver experiences symptoms of **sleep depravation.** Even when they do get some sleep, it may not be a restful sleep, because they are trying to listen for the senior, in case assistance is needed.

Before the caregiver starts to wear out, it may be time to look for other alternatives. It is natural that the main focus of **visitors** is for the patient, but **don't forget the caregiver**. **CaregiverStress.com** offers free monthly seminars for family caregivers on subjects such as nutrition, managing medications, stress, finances, and managing sibling dynamics.

The more other family members get involved, the better. That includes young **children.** The children can help with small tasks, depending upon their age. When our children were in elementary school, my mother-in-law was ill and not able to care for herself at home, so we took her into our home. Our children helped by running small errands for her, or spending time visiting with her and keeping her company. That experience helped them develop a closer relationship with her, and even helped prepare them for her eventual death.

CHAPTER XIV

SKILLED NURSING FACILITIES

There have always been many misconceptions, regarding nursing homes, that make many people dread the idea of having to be admitted to one. I remember when I was a child, 65 years ago, the dread was that if you ever had to go to a nursing home, you never left there alive.

Today nursing homes, now called **Skilled Nursing Facilities (SNF)**, are much different than they were in the 1940s. When I was a nursing student, if anyone asked me if I would work in a nursing home, I would have answered a definite "no". But a few years after I graduated, I did take a position in a nursing home and loved working there. That was in the early 1960s and even then, they were spending a great deal of time focusing on rehabilitation. Rather than the nursing home being a place for people to stay until they died, it became a place where people could be rehabilitated and return home.

Skilled nursing facilities (SNF) still provide a place for someone to spend their **final days,** but more often it provides **temporary skilled care,** until the individuals are well enough to return home. Hence the name "Skilled Nursing Facilities". Some of these changes are related to advances in our ability for rehabilitation following injuries, surgeries, and medical conditions, such as strokes.

Additionally, because of early discharges from medical centers, some individuals may need extended nursing care or therapy before they are able to return home. Because of the admission of more acutely ill patients to SNFs, the caliber of their staff has improved.

We think of SNFs as a place for the elderly, but you will, also, find some younger patients. Most often those patients are victims of severe disabilities, such as spinal cord injuries or a degenerative disease, such as Multiple Sclerosis.

The **quality of care** in most SNFs has improved in recent decades. They **must meet certain standards** in order to maintain their **licensure** to operate in their states, and also, to receive reimbursement from **Medicare and Medicaid.** Some of the high quality SNFs are also accredited, which means they must meet even more stringent standards.

Skilled Nursing Facilities strive to provide a comfortable atmosphere for the residents. It is recognized that many of their "customers" are there as a permanent resident. Therefore, they are referred to as residents. Most SNFs have **resident/family counsels,** and everyone is encouraged to participate. Additionally, the staff tries to meet with residents and/or family on a regular basis to **review the resident's care plan.**

Some facilities are now being designed to provide a more **resident friendly setting**. These facilities are arranged in small groups of 10-30 residents, who share a small kitchen, communal area, and the same staff. One advantage of this setting is a staff who is familiar with the residents, and the residents have an opportunity to get to know and trust the staff.

Services may vary according to the payers which reimburse for the residents care. Also, some SNFs **specialize** in certain areas of care, such as rehabilitation or dementia care.

One of the **main third party payers** for SNFs is Medicare. A facility that wants to receive reimbursement from **Medicare and/or Medicaid** is required to have **licensed practical nurses** on duty 24 hours a day, and a **registered nurse** on duty at least 8 hours per day, 7 days a week.

Medicare provides up to **100 days** of care, when there is documentation of a **need for skilled care.** The amount of Medicare coverage does vary during those 100 days. The first 20 days are fully covered. The remaining days are covered, but require a co-payment.

Skilled care includes nursing and rehabilitation care. Some examples of **skilled nursing** are wound care and intravenous therapy. **Skilled rehabilitation** includes physical, occupational, and speech-language therapy. For more details, go to **www.CMS.gov (Centers for Medicare & Medicaid Services)** This web site provides full details of SNF coverage.

Medicaid covers basic **custodial care,** such as activities of daily living for residents who are eligible for Medicaid coverage. Someone who is exploring the option of Medicaid eligibility might want to **consult an attorney,** who specializes in elder law. **Medical social workers** can also be helpful in exploring the eligibility requirements and how they are achieved.

It is helpful to contact your local Medicaid office. As I found, when inquiring about options for my elderly cousin, the individual may not be eligible for Medicaid, but there could be other options available for assistance.

REMINDER: I strongly urge people to purchase some type of **long-term care insurance**. The earlier in life that the insurance is purchased, the cheaper the premiums will be.

Private pay for nursing homes, at this time, runs about $5000 per month. One can see that it wouldn't take much time for a person's savings to be wiped out, if the resident needs care for an indefinite period of time for something like dementia. Besides help in paying for the bills, insurance companies have more **clout to negotiate** better rates for the resident.

Guidelines for Making a Decision When Choosing a Care Facility.

First you have to **decide** which **type of facility** would meet your needs best. It may be helpful to include all immediate family members or friends, who may be directly involved in the patient's life. For sure, the **patient** should be **involved in** the **decision making** as much as possible, even if the individual is very ill or may have dementia. The more informed the person is, the more cooperative they will be when it is time to make a move.

It is wise to **discuss these issues early**, before one gets gets to the point when the decision must be made. I have seen situations where the family has gone ahead and made major decisions without involving the senior. It created unnecessary problems and unrest within the family. Some of these problems created a rift that was never resolved, even after the death of the senior.

I do suggest that close family members, who do not live nearby, be kept involved. If you are that family member who lives a distance away, it will be beneficial for you to be supportive of the decisions that are made and keep in close contact with the senior and other family members. Of course, all of this will depend upon the closeness of relationships within the family.

Home care may still be an option with the use of additional assistance. Most seniors do prefer to stay at home, so if it is possible for them to to do so without adding unreasonable stress to the rest of the family, that may be the best option.

Safety is a major factor that must be considered when making a decision. When dementia is involved, safety becomes even more of an issue.

The **next** step, after it is decided the senior needs more care than what is possible at home, is to determine which facility can best provide that care. In recent years, there has been an increase in the availability of retirement and assisted living facilities.

One **major factor** that influences the decision would be the **senior's condition**.

- Is it temporary?
- Will it get worse?
- How much disability is involved?
- Does the senior just need custodial care or is there a need for skilled care?

Other factors are the senior's preferences and whether money is an issue.

Retirement facilities usually provide private **apartments, meals, van service, activities, and housekeeping services.** This may be sufficient support to meet the needs of the senior. Many people, on a fixed income, have found they are able to afford living in a retirement home, especially if you consider that food and utilities are covered in the rent. Also, seniors have found they have opportunities for more social contacts, than when they were living at home.

Assisted Living facilities provide the next level of care for seniors. These facilities usually have the **same services as offered in a retirement home,** and additionally, provide help with **activities of daily living,** such as bathing, dressing, transferring from bed to chair, and walking. There are some facilities that provide both retirement and assisted living levels of help. The next chapter will discuss these two types of facilities in more detail.

When it is apparent that a **Skilled Nursing Facility** is needed, the next step is to decide which SNF is best suited for the senior. It is highly recommended to **take time to visit** the facilities that are being considered. Hopefully, the senior will be well enough to also make the visits. If there is still a question between choosing an assisted living facility and an SNF, it would be helpful to visit both types of facilities.

You may find it helpful to refer to **"Nursing Home Compare" at www.medicare.gov,** when making a decision. This web site provides useful information about all the SNFs in your area. There are, also, similar sites that allow you to compare other healthcare resources, such as medical centers, physicians, and home health agencies.

The nursing home web site allows you to **compare up to three facilities at a time.** It gives you an overall rating of the facilities related to **health inspections, staffing, and quality measures.** It, also, indicates the number of beds in each facility, if they participate in Medicare and Medicaid, and if it is a profit or nonprofit corporation.

Besides the overall ratings, this program allows you to see more details related to this evaluation, including details about **health inspections, staffing, and quality measures.** This information will help you decide what questions will be important to ask when you visit these facilities. It will, also, help you prioritize which facilities you will want to visit.

Another resource, that can help you make a decision, is the **local long-term care ombudsmen.** They visit these facilities and can give you guidance on which facilities might best meet the needs of your elder member.

Within the booklet, **Medicare Coverage of Skilled Nursing Facility Care** (www.**cms.gov**), there is a Skilled Nursing Facility **Checklist** you may find helpful when you are making your visits. You may not want to use that specific format, but it will give you some ideas of what information is important for you obtain.

Be sure to **make appointments** for your visits. Most facilities have a designated person to provide tours for prospective residents. Take with you a **list of questions** you will want to ask at each facility. Be sure to include questions related to the specific needs of your prospective resident.

Suggested questions and observations to help you choose a facility:
Facility:

- Does it look **clean**? comfortable? cluttered? pleasant? inviting? homelike? well-lit? noisy?
- How does it **smell**?
- Does it seem **secure**? Are there smoke detectors, sprinklers, handrails in hallways, and grab bars in bathrooms?
- What do the **residents' rooms** look like? How much space do they have?
- Can they have some of their own belongings? a piece of their **own furniture**? pictures? bedspread?

- Do they have adequate **storage space**?
- Do the rooms look **bright**? **cheerful**?
- Do they have access to a personnel phone, computer, and TV?

Staff:

- What is the **rate of staff turnover?** Include the turnover rate of the **administrator** and director of nurses (**DON**)?
- What are the staffing levels, including for nights and weekends?
- Do you **feel welcome**?
- Do they seem interested in you and your senior? (That is one of the advantages of bringing the potential resident. You can observe how they interact with each other.)
- Do they all wear **name tags** that are easy to read?
- Do they introduce themselves and their role?
- How do they **interact with the current residents?** Do they know their names?
- (Most of these facilities are small enough and most of the residents are there long enough that even the DON should know the residents.)
- **How knowledgeable** are they about your resident's condition?
- How often does the **staff** receive **training?**

- What is the **staffing ratio** per resident? (Don't just note numbers but also levels of staff, i.e. number of RNs and LPNs to supervise aides.)
- Do the residents tend to receive care from the **same group** of staff?

Medical care:

- Who provides the medical care? Is there a **licensed physician** on staff?
- How frequently is the resident medical care plan evaluated. (There should be an increased frequency, if the resident is receiving skilled care.)
- Can they still see their own physician?

Residents:

- Do they **look clean?** comfortable? well groomed?
- What is the bathing and grooming routines?
- Do **room lights** seem to be answered in a timely manner?
- Are there family members and friends visiting? You might **ask them** how they and their resident like the facility.
- Are **personal belongings respected** by the staff?
- Do they have a choice for **roommates?**
- Are there **quiet, pleasant areas for visits** with family and friends?

- Do residents get a **choice of foods**?
- Do they **receive help** with their meals?
- Do they receive nutritious snacks?
- Is there an active **resident/family council** with regular meetings?

Activities:

- Do they involve most of the residents? (It is helpful to be able to **observe** an **activity session** and schedule.)
- Is exercise included in the activity schedule?
- How are the activities advertised?
- Are there outdoor activities?
- Are there **extra amenities**, such as a beauty salon, available?

Experience with special needs:

- How does the facility handle **wanderers**?
- Does it provide for **special programs** needed by your resident?
- Is the facility secure?
- Is there a system to keep track of all residents?
- How are **medications and treatments** handled?

Other:

- Are they **Medicare and/or Medicaid approved?**
- Are recent **state inspection reports** posted?

- What is the monthly **cost**?
- What are the **extra charges**? (Frequently personal laundry, medications, equipment use, incontinent pads, and other supplies cost extra.)
- How flexible are the visiting hours?

REMINDER: Before making a final decision, it might be wise to make another **unannounced visit.** Just to make sure your observations of the facility are consistent.

When the facility has been selected and your resident has been admitted, be sure to **keep in close contact,** so the resident does not feel abandoned. Hopefully, someone lives close enough to be able to visit fairly frequently. It is wise to **visit at different times** of the day to get a feel for the kind of care that is provided throughout the day. Frequent visits also help you get to know all the staff.

You can expect that there will be a **period of adjustment** for the new resident. It would not be unusual for the resident to experience some depression. That is where friends and family can be especially helpful. Don't get upset if they do have **complaints.** It helps them to be able to express their feelings. You might be able to problem solve some of their complaints. Other complaints might be easily solved by involving the nursing staff.

NEVER dismiss the resident's complaints without investigating, even if they have dementia. They may be providing some important information. You are their main advocate.

You can also **help your resident get involved** in activities which may hasten their adjustment. If you live far away, plan to keep in touch via phone and letters. **Cheerful and colorful cards** are always helpful. Be sure the staff knows how to reach the designated contact person and encourage them to call. If they know you are involved, they will be more inclined to keep in touch with you.

It is important for the family to **keep in contact with** the resident's **physician**. Do not hesitate to ask questions. Usually physicians do not visit their SNF patients more than once a month.

Some physicians turn the care of their patients over to the **SNF medical staff.** Hopefully, you will know that before you select an SNF, and will have an opportunity to meet the medical staff. The resident's physician may still be willing to check in on them, from time to time.

Getting involved in the **resident/family council** is important and, also, encourage your resident to get involved. That is, also, an opportunity to get to know other residents and their families. It keeps you aware of special issues that affect SNFs. If you are not able to participate in the council meetings, take opportunities to visit with other residents and family members.

Also keep in contact with the **local ombudsman.** Most SNFs will review resident rights on admission, but if you need more details, the ombudsman is a good resource.

I found that I could save my cousin some money by taking her **personal laundry** home to wash. I was also able to keep track of her belongings that way. There were times when some of her clothes ended up in her roommate's closet, so I was able to retrieve them or return her roommate's clothes, that mistakenly landed in Em's closet. I also **purchased** her **a wheelchair,** which paid for itself several times over from what she saved on the facility's rental fees .

Finally, keep in mind that if you and the resident are not happy there, after allowing for a reasonable adjustment period, you do not have to stay there. **You do have the option to move**.

It is also your **right to change physicians.** Before you do, it is wise to make sure that you have another physician willing to take over the care.

CHAPTER XV

SENIOR RETIREMENT & ASSISTED LIVING FACILITIES

Today, there are many options available for the elderly, faced with physical limitations related to aging, who are no longer able to safely live alone in their homes. There may be confusion over what services are offered by each type of facility.

Facilities for seniors who are still relatively independent may be referred to by a variety of different titles. Some titles are: Independent Living, Retirement Community/ Facility, or Senior Apartment Facility.

Retirement Communities are usually groups of homes, condos, or mobile homes for people 55 years or older, that provide yard maintenance and recreation centers. These are beneficial for seniors who want to down size, and desire opportunities to socialize. There is, also, subsidized senior housing, for low income seniors, that fit into this category.

Retirement Facilities usually provide individual apartments for the residents. Additionally, transportation, meals in a general dining room, and housekeeping services are provided. The residents are able to live independently, but the facilities will still keep track of them in case of an emergency. Usually, each apartment will have a call system that can be used in case of an emergency. Resident Facilities provide an option for individuals who are generally independent, but are better off not driving and have difficulty keeping up with housekeeping and cooking. These facilities usually do provide parking for those residents who still have their own cars.

Assisted Living and Board and Care Homes provide more personal care for individuals who need assistance with activities of daily living. These facilities are more closely regulated by the individual states.

Assisted Living facilities may provide individual apartments, rooms, or shared rooms. **Board and Care homes** tend to be smaller facilities or residences that provide care to a limited number of residents. Many Board and Care facilities provide a comfortable, homelike atmosphere. Both of these types of facilities will usually provide **personal care, ambulation assistance, meals, and assistance with eating,** as needed. They will also assist with medical care the residents would normally do for themselves, such as **medication administration**. The staff, in these facilities, must complete **additional training** to assist with medications. The staff is available **24 hours a day.**

There are some facilities that provide a **combination of Residence and Assisted Living** services. This type of facility can make it convenient for individuals who anticipate they may need more assistance in the future. The assisted living services are usually billed separately, depending upon what services are rendered.

Some communities, also, offer **Continuing Care Retirement Communities (CCRC).** Their housing may be apartments, condos, or individual houses. They offer **different levels of care,** including Retirement, Assisted Living, and Nursing Home. These communities charge an **entry fee** (which may be a large payment), in addition to **monthly rent.** Some of these communities may provide an option for the members to purchase their residence.

When considering the possibility of joining this type of community, one needs to **investigate the Skilled Nursing Facility (SNF),** in case that level of care is ever needed. Some of these SNFs are only available to the CCRC'S members. Members of these communities can usually move from the retirement level of care to the assisted level, without having to change their current residence.

Guidelines for Choosing a Facility: Research various facility options:

- Which type of facility meets your present and future needs?
- Which facility has expertise in dealing with your physical or mental condition?
- Which facilities are available in your community?
- Are they in a safe area and close to family and friends?
- What is the cost?

- Be aware that these facilities may change ownership.
- Make sure the contract you end up signing will protect you, even with a change in ownership.
- If you have Long-Term Care Insurance, is this type of facility covered?
- If receiving any State or Federal assistance, would this facility qualify?
- What is the occupancy rate of the facility? (Sometimes you can spot a problem, i.e. a rapid turnover of residents.)
- Seek input from State regulating agencies and the local ombudsman.
- Review suggestions for choosing a Skilled Nursing Facility in chapter XIV.

Consider Individual Preferences:

- What is your income?
- What are your needs and priorities? (Transportation, recreation, socialization, assistance with activities of daily living, help with meals and housekeeping.)

Visit facilities of interest:

- Most of these facilities are happy to have visitors.
- Do you feel welcome?

- Take a written list of questions you want answered.

Meals:

- If the facility offers communal meals, it is helpful to accept an invitation to a meal. (It gives you an opportunity to assess the meals and see many of the residents.)
- When are meals served?
- Is there a dress code?
- Any other rules for the dinning room?

Tour:

- Is there a pleasant atmosphere?
- Is the facility clean?
- Does the staff seem friendly and helpful?
- What is the cost?
- Does the contract have limits on how rapidly the rent can be raised?
- Are there extra charges for personal services?
- Are there safety features? (Outside door kept locked? Security alarms? Hand rails in hallways? Grab bars in bathrooms and showers? Call bells in apartments/ rooms, especially in bathrooms?)

Visit with the residents.

- Are they friendly?

- Do they seem happy with the facility?
- Is there an active resident council?
- Is the staff open to meeting with and working with the council?
- What does the activity schedule look like?
- Is there a variety of activities?
- What is your impression of the activity facilities?
- Is everything located conveniently?
- Are the apartments or rooms pleasant? (Sufficient space?)
- What are the policies regarding personal belongings?
- Do they accommodate wheelchairs and walkers?
- Any there restrictions on visitors?

Van Transportation:

- What are the rules regarding transportation?
- Are rides provided to church, for medical appointments, and for shopping?

Planning an unannounced visit, before making a final decision, can be helpful.

When the Facility is chosen:

- Document apartment condition when moving in and, again, when moving out. (Photos are helpful).

- Allow time for adjustment to changes. (Keep in mind adjustment will not happen overnight.)
- Keep in contact with family and friends.
- Get involved within the facility.
- If able, attend council meetings and participate in activities.
- Stay active.
- When moving out, arrange an inspection by facility manager to avoid unexpected   damage charges.

Assisted Living Services:
When receiving extra services:

- Keep track of the number of visits and length of time for each visit.
- Make sure the charges are consistent with the services rendered.
- There should be a supervisor visiting, from time to time, to make sure you are receiving the proper care.
- If you have any questions about your care, do not hesitate to call the office of the supervisor.
- Do not leave money or valuables, such as jewelry, laying around. (Most people providing these services are honest, but occasionally, you may find someone who is dishonest.)

- Keep track of your checkbook. (My cousin had some checks stolen out of the back of her checkbook, which she did not notice, until one of those checks was cashed,)
- Many facilities provide safes in the resident rooms/ apartments. If you have one, make use of it.

CHAPTER XVI

ELDER GUARDIANSHIP OR MANAGEMENT

This step should never be taken lightly. After we have spent a major part of our lives determining our own destinies, it is difficult giving up freedom, even if we realize that it needs to happen.

It is always best to **plan ahead,** rather than waiting until you are forced to make changes. Make sure your family and/or close friends **know your wishes.** Then make sure you put your wishes **in writing,** especially whom you designate to handle your affairs and make decisions for you, if you become incapacitated or die. This can help avoid lengthily and expensive court hearings and can, also, help avoid family disputes.

There are different terms that may be used to imply elder guardianship or management. These terms may vary regarding the legal degree of the guardian's responsibility and the state of residence of the elder.

The term **guardianship** (conservatorship or fiduciaries) usually implies a **court appointed** responsibility. Some **less formal terms** that may be used are **advocate, manager, or agent.** Some elder managers and advocates are specially trained and charge a fee. However, family members or friends may act in these capacities.

An **advocate** is one who acts as a liaison between the elder and health care providers or other types of agencies, the elder may encounter. An advocate may be a **family member, friend, or a health care provider,** such as a nurse or other professional. There are **some organizations** that may, also, provide advocacy services, such as the Alzheimer's Association or the American Cancer Society. The advocacy may be a temporary process or may be ongoing, depending upon the needs of the elder.

If you are the one who is taking on the role of the guardian or agent, you need to be **sensitive and understanding** of the one who will be losing some independence. I remember when my mother-in-law was signing papers to have my husband be a cosigner on her checking account. She had a difficult time signing the forms, even though she knew it was the right thing to do and she knew that my husband could be trusted. As she pointed out, it would be just the **first step** of gradually having to give up her independence and control.

This brings up the importance for elder individuals to be sure to **choose agents** that can be trusted to be responsible and look out for their best interests. The individual taking on guardianship needs to keep the elder informed and encourage participation in the decision making, as appropriate. Even someone with dementia needs to be kept informed of changes that may be directly affecting them.

I knew **two elderly sisters,** who were both in their 80s. They shared an apartment and helped take care of each other. They were both mentally competent. Their family was concerned about them because they lived in a different state from most of their relatives. So the family made arrangements, without consulting the sisters, to move them 2000 miles away. The sisters were informed of the move a month before they were to leave. The move turned out to be so traumatic that one sister died shortly after the move.

The other sister ended up feeling she was "stuck" in the new state. I am happy to report she was finally able to get back to her original state. She phoned us when she got back and talked about how happy she was to be home. Sadly, she had lost a lot of her personal possessions that family members had either sold or given away, when she originally moved. The family was well meaning, but unfortunately, they forgot to include the two sisters in their decision making. If these two elderly ladies had been involved from the beginning, I feel the outcome could have been much better for them.

When my cousin became disabled, she knew she would need to move closer to someone who could help her. She had been a single lady all her life, but she had kept close contact with several relatives. Her example reminded me of the **importance of keeping in touch** and helping others, because you never know when you will need their help. When she decided she wanted to move close to us, it was apparent she was going to have to **downsize** her possessions. We **moved slowly**, sorting out what would be moved with her, what would be given away, and what would be sold.

This, also, gave me an **opportunity to become more familiar with her wishes.**

Decisions for guardianship need to be **individualized.** I have seen families who work well together and share decisions regarding their parents. There are, also, families that can not be trusted to make even the most minor decision, on behalf of their parents. There are some situations where it works to have two people share the guardianship responsibilities, whereas, there are other times it works best to have one person be designated as the guardian. It would be ideal, if the **designated person** be one who lives in the **same community** as the elder. It helps if the legal documents specify the responsibilities of each person. In the case of a **guardianship**, the court does specify the responsibilities and limitations of the guardian. Not only does the elder need to be kept informed, but the people sharing the responsibilities need to keep each other informed.

There are many times when the elder does not have a family member or friend who can take on or be trusted with the responsibilities of guardianship. In such cases, the **court system** may have to step in when the elders can no longer manage their own affairs. In such situations, states have defined a **hierarchy** of who is eligible to take over as the guardian, especially if there is a sudden event that renders the elder unable to make decisions. This process tends to be expensive and difficult. If you are someone who **does not have immediate family members,** you can save time and extra expenses by **designating in writing a trusted friend** who is willing and able to take on this role.

Confidentiality is a major concern when someone is functioning as a guardian. The elder has every **right to privacy**. The guardian or agent is likely to become privy to information, concerning the elder, that would not be available otherwise. Professionals are obligated, legally and ethically, to maintain confidentially, whereas, an agent may not necessarily be bound to the same legal restraints. It is more a **moral issue** for the agent. The agent needs to think about how they would want their own personal information handled. A court appointed guardian is expected to maintain confidentiality. Find out with whom and what information the elder would want shared. Of course, it is best that if dementia is not involved, to **let the elder decide what they want to share** and when they choose to share.

REMINDER: A good guideline for confidentiality is asking the question: Does this person/agency have the right to the information and do they need it?

Advocate for respect. When I would accompany my cousin to an appointment, some people would just talk to me and not to her. She did not have a hearing problem and was very capable of making her own decisions. I was there to help her interpret the medical information, not to make her decisions. I would tactfully redirect the attention back to her. There are some people who make assumptions that an elderly person is not capable of understanding what is happening. My cousin used to laugh because people would assume that she could not hear. She used to pick up more gossip that way.

The **next chapter** will have a more detailed discussion of legal documents that may be helpful for that time in your life when you are no longer able to handle your own affairs and prepare for end of life.

CHAPTER XVII

ADVANCED DIRECTIVES

Advanced Directive is a term which indicates documents used to record individuals' wishes regarding medical care in the event they are no longer able to make decisions, due to illness or incapacity. Some of these documents are commonly know as a **Living Will, Power Of Attorney (POA),** and **Do Not Resuscitate (DNR)**.

The **Living Will** provides detailed instructions about medical care to be carried out if individuals are unable to voice their wishes. It is helpful to include in the document any **circumstances that would trigger** these measures, e.g., "in the event of an incurable illness or condition".

Some Living Wills are very general and simply indicate that the individual does not want extreme measures taken, if their condition indicates there is no hope for recovery. Other Living Wills are more specific and indicate what measures the individual wishes **NOT** to receive and which ones should **CONTINUE** to be administered. Some of these **measures could include** cardiopulmonary resuscitation (CPR), breathing tube, kidney dialysis, feeding tube, food and water, or the use of a ventilator. The Living Will may, also, specify that antibiotics, hydration, and pain measures should continue to be used. They may contain special directions in case of death, such as permission to **donate organs**.

There are forms available that provide **guidelines** for the individual to use when filling out these documents. The forms are designed so that one can express how much or how little is to be done, when one can no longer make decisions.

A **Durable Medical Power Of Attorney** is used to indicate a **health care proxy** who will make health care decisions for an individual, if that person becomes incapacitated and unable to make decisions. Other terms that may be used to refer to the proxy are **attorney-in-fact, surrogate, or agent.** Some terms used for the individual being represented are **principal or grantor.** Some of **these terms vary** in accordance with an individual state. It is wise to **consult** a **lawyer** familiar with local state requirements for these documents.

There are **different types** of Power Of Attorney (POA) forms. It is wise to fill out **both** main types; **Medical** Power Of Attorney and **Financial** Power Of Attorney. Some people may want to have one person handle medical decisions and another handle the financial decisions. Others may have one individual handle both areas.

A POA can be written in a **general** way or in a **limited** fashion that puts limits on the scope of the proxy's responsibilities. A **Durable** Power Of Attorney is used to insure the POA continues even if the grantor becomes incapacitated.

Another type of advanced directive is a **Do Not Resuscitate (DNR).** Most medical facilities will ask patients if they want a DNR, especially if they already have a Living Will or Medical Power Of Attorney. If someone has signed a DNR, medical professionals will interpret that to mean the individual does **NOT** want **cardiopulmonary resuscitation (CPR)** in the event they should stop breathing or their heart should stop.

The DNR will usually imply that the individual would NOT want to be **intubated** (insertion of a breathing tube) nor placed on a **ventilator** (breathing machine). Some states require that a signed **DNI (Do Not Intubate)** be included with the DNR.

Frequently, people who choose to sign a DNR are ones who have a **terminal disease** with little or no hope of recovery. Examples would be someone with terminal cancer, chronic lung disease, chronic kidney disease, or someone in a permanent unconscious state.

Just because someone has a signed a Living Will or Durable Power of Attorney, it **does not mean** that they do not want to be resuscitated. Even if they indicate in their living will that they want a DNR, it is advised they, also, **sign a DNR/DNI,** which is usually signed by their doctor as well. That document then becomes part of the medical orders.

If for some reason, resuscitation of an individual who has a signed DNR does take place because the medical personnel were not aware of the document, it does not mean the individual must remain on a respirator or continue to be intubated. Those measures **can be reversed** by the physician, once the document or individual's wishes are verified by the agent with Medical Power of Attorney.

An Advanced Directive does not mean that the individual cannot receive any medical treatment. The individual is **still entitled** to comfort and pain relief. Even if the individual has a terminal disease and they should fall and injure themselves, they are entitled to receive treatment for their injuries.

It, also, does not mean that once the document is signed, you cannot **change your mind**. A DNR/DNI may be revoked at any time by the principal, as long as that individual is mentally competent. It can be done **verbally,** but is always best to follow up with a new written document.

There are **standardized forms and guidelines** available for the different types of Advanced Directives. Resources include lawyers' offices and state government web sites; to name a couple. It is wise to obtain a form that is approved by the state of residence. To qualify as a legal document, it must be signed. Additionally, some states require a witnessed signature, that may also need to be notarized.

Be sure to check these documents from time to time to make sure they are **up-to-date**. (For example, my cousin had a detailed trust made out, but the executor she designated had died.) You may also change your mind about how much medical intervention you want in the event you have a medical emergency.

If there is no Advanced Directive, each state designates a **priority list** of who might make medical decisions, in case the individual is no longer capable of doing so. Usually the spouse would be the primary decision maker or a parent for a minor. This fact reinforces the **importance** of a **written advanced directive,** especially for someone who may not be married or is estranged from their spouse.

REMINDER: Make sure you **share** copies of your Living Will, Medical Power Of Attorney, and DNR with your immediate family and/or close friend(s), so in a time of emergency, everyone will be aware of your wishes.

If you are an agent or surrogate, you **cannot be held liable** for any decisions you have made on behalf of that person, nor for any expenses accrued, as long as you are acting within the authority of the POA. It can be daunting enough to make these decisions without having to worry about a liability.

From personal experience, I learned that these decisions are far easier to make if the person's wishes are known beforehand. It is very wise to **keep clear records** about any decisions made and/or actions taken on behalf of the principal's wishes. A **short narrative** about the circumstances and why those decisions were made will also be helpful.

It is, also, wise to keep others who are close to the individual informed, but remember to **respect the principle's privacy.** (I was careful to ensure that I had my cousin's permission to share information.)

REMINDER: Be sure to notify the principal's primary medical provider, bank, lawyer, care facility, government agency, etc., that you are the individual's designated Power Of Attorney. These establishments will probably request a copy of the POA.

All of these documents can be comprehensively organized as part of an **Estate Plan**. An up-to-date estate plan can help heirs avoid an expensive and time-consuming probate process. The key word is "up-to-date". Assistance obtaining literature, forms, and guidelines for all of these documents can be obtained from a local lawyer, at a library, and on the internet. Some **recommended web sites** are state and federal government sites. There are, also, several legal and medical sites that provide individualized assistance and advice.

REMINDER: You can save your heirs extra concern by purchasing **burial/funeral insurance** for when the time comes. (I made sure my cousin's funeral and burial expenses were taken care of, before all her money was used up for nursing home expenses.)

CHAPTER XVIII

END-OF-LIFE CARE

End-of-Life care refers to the placing of the main focus of care on relief of pain and other end-of-life issues. It does not necessarily mean that curative measures will no longer be used.

Some examples of conditions that could prompt an end of life focus are:

- **Terminal illness,** like end stage kidney disease or cancer.
- **Chronic conditions,** like chronic lung or cardiac disease.
- **Degenerative diseases,** like multiple sclerosis.
- **Cognitive conditions,** like alzheimer's disease.

We don't always like having to think about dying, but this is a **time to plan and make decisions** that need to be made before we do die. It, also, could provide an opportunity to resolve and/or bring closure to some issues and relationships.

This period of time may last for a few weeks or years. The focus for end-of-life care tends to develop when individuals, along with their families, start to **realize** they are **not getting better** and the treatment no longer seems to be working. This may be the time when individuals decide they would

prefer being at home, rather than spending their final days in a hospital or undergoing extensive treatments.

Hopefully, most decisions regarding end-of-life care have already been made. It would be ideal if financial arrangements have been made, so finances do not have to add to an already stressful situation. These decisions often depend upon how the individual and family usually cope with grief.

Grief is often experienced in different stages. The most common stages observed include **shock/denial** (It can't be), **bargaining** (I just need a little more time), **depression** (I can hardly face the day), **anger** (Why did this have to happen to me), and **acceptance** (OK, I will get ready).

Many dying people, stated they did experience these five stages, but not necessarily in the same order. Additionally, not all people experience all five stages.

Family members and others who surround dying individuals, including professional and nonprofessional care givers, can, also, experience the stages of grief. It is believed that these stages are encountered, not only with terminal illness, but as well with other losses such as loss of a body part, divorce, or job loss. Frequently, people move back and forth between these different stages, when they are dealing with grief.

It helps to know that these symptoms are common, so you realize there is nothing wrong with you or your loved one. The individual, with a terminal illness, **needs to be**

supported when dealing with their loss, no matter which stage of grief they happen to be experiencing.

Frequently, we may feel uncomfortable being around someone who is dying because we do not know what to say or are afraid we might say the wrong thing. Dying patients are more **fearful** of being **abandoned** or being a **burden.** You don't need to worry about what to say to the patient; just taking some time to **sit with** them helps. Also, letting them know you are there to **listen** if they want to talk, will give them comfort.

Hospice services can provide valuable resources for terminally ill individuals and their families. Hospice is a type of philosophy of care for those dealing with a terminal illness. It involves a **full system of care** focused to **alleviate physical**, **emotional,** and **social** symptoms experienced by the dying individual.

A **team of professionals,** including doctors, nurses, therapists, social workers, and non professionals (nursing assistants and housekeepers), work together to meet the patient's needs. The **focus** of care **moves from** trying to cure the illness to providing **palliative care** to alleviate the **symptoms** of the condition, including pain relief.

The **concept of hospice** is traced back to the time of the crusades. Hospices were established to care for the incurably ill. The care was provided by the crusaders. Additionally, hospices were used to provide shelter for travelers.

In 1967, physician **Dame Cicely Saunders** created the first modern hospice in London. In 1974, an associate of Dame Saunders, Florence Wald, Dean of Yale School of Nursing, established the first hospice in the United States,

Today, most people receiving hospice services are at **home** and cared for by family or friends. When patients are cared for at home, they have more opportunity to **control** their own care. However, people can receive hospice services at **skilled nursing facilities** or hospice **inpatient facilities,** that are Medicare approved. The hospice agency, providing the services at home, must also, be **Medicare approved.**

Room and board charges, in a facility, are **not usually covered** under hospice services. One could have those charges covered through a separate long term care insurance policy, or if they are covered by Medicaid.

Medicare will pay for hospice services for those who are eligible for Medicare Part A services. Many private insurances will, also, cover hospice care.

Medicare rules for hospice services include:
1. Certification from 2 physicians who verify that the individual is expected to live 6 months or less, if their disease runs it's normal course. The two physicians usually would include the individual's personal physician and the medical director for the hospice agency. (A nurse practitioner cannot be one of the certifiers.)

This rule does not mean that if one lives longer than 6 months they can no longer receive hospice care, but it does mean that they need to be **recertified.** As long as the physicians agree that the individual continues to be terminal, they may be recertified several times.

The recertification process may require some extra time on the part of the patient and family, from time to time. It is helpful to be cooperative. The agency is required to perform recertifications on a regular basis, in order to maintain eligibility for reimbursement for services.

2. It is expected that the individual will **no longer receive life saving treatment,** such as chemotherapy for cancer. However, **cancer** is not the only condition that makes someone eligible for hospice services. People in the **end stage** of **heart, lung, and kidney** diseases or **degenerative** diseases can also benefit from hospice.

This rule does not mean one could not receive other medical treatment for conditions not related to the terminal illness, such as a broken bone or an infection. The **medical care** for conditions **not related** to the terminal disease, including emergency room care, must be given or **arranged for by the hospice medical team** in order to be reimbursed by Medicare.

REMINDER: Be sure to contact the hospice agency before:

- Using the ambulance.
- Going to the emergency room or urgent care facility.
- Arranging for medical treatment not related to the terminal illness.

3. If the patient decides not to **continue hospice** so another therapy can be tried, the patient is welcome to do so. In that situation, Medicare patients would revert back to the Medicare coverage they had before going on hospice. Later, if the new treatment is not effective and the physicians determine the patient is terminal, hospice may be reinitiated.

Hospice services that will be covered by Medicare includes:

1. Hospice team services which includes physician, nursing, therapy (physical, occupational, speech-language), social services, dietary, and counseling.

2. An individualized plan of care developed by the professional staff, based on medical data and the professional staff's assessments. The more candid the patient and family are, the better the care plan will be for meeting the patient's needs.

3. Hospice **aide** and **homemaker** services.

4. Prescription drugs ordered for control of symptoms. (Drugs used to cure the illness will not be covered.) A copayment may be required for all types of drugs.

5. Medical equipment (wheelchair, walker) and medical **supplies** (dressings, catheters).

6. Other services needed for pain and symptom control.

7. Short-term inpatient or respite care, arranged by the hospice team, to provide some relief for the caregiver. There may be a small copayment that the patient/family will have to pay. (Room and board will not be covered if the individual is a **full-time patient** in a nursing home or hospice facility.)

All these **supplies and services** need to be reflected on the patient's plan of care and justified in the patient record.

Most hospices will utilize **part-time** and/or **volunteer staff.** Some of this staff may have expertise in certain areas, such as **legal** or **religious**, to help patients and families make decisions about estate planning, **funeral planning,** or other complex end of life decisions.

Other volunteers assist with **respite** and other services, such as housekeeping or counseling. Hospice organizations have **special training for the volunteers** to help them work with the special needs of terminal patients and their families, especially concerning loss.

Many hospice agencies receive **additional support through donations.** They, also, may have a **thrift shop** to raise extra money. Some hospice agencies have **equipment** (walkers, hospital beds) and **supplies** (wigs, dressings) available for use by their clients.

Hospice agencies provide **24/7 availability of medical and nursing staff** for support and service. The hospice services provide support and care throughout the course of the patient's illness, including at the **time of death and death aftercare**.

Usually, there will be a **registered nurse** who oversees and coordinates the care. This person will be the best person to contact if there are any problems or questions. Even if that person is not the one with the needed expertise, they can arrange for the right one to handle the issue. The agency will leave **information in the home** to use in case of a problem. You are not expected to wait until someone makes a visit or until the problem becomes an emergency to call the office.

If you happen to know that your case manager is off, you can still **call the office** for help. There will always be someone available to help you.

Do not try to contact your case manager directly during off hours, or if your case manager is on vacation. Always **call the office**. We had one situation where the patient needed help and left a message on the nurse's cell phone. The nurse was out of town for a few days and did not get the message until she returned. Fortunately, this instance was not an emergency, but the patient could have had the problem solved much sooner, if the office had been called rather than the nurse.

The plan of care **focuses on the whole person** including physical, mental, spiritual, emotional, cultural, and social needs. While receiving hospice services, if you feel you are not receiving the support and care you need, do not hesitate to tell them. This includes support needed when dealing with loss.

Usually, by the time death is eminent, the patient has a **Do Not Resuscitate,** however, this is not a requirement for hospice services.

Frequently, patients desire to die at home unless they feel they have become too much of a burden. If you are the caregiver or family member of the individual, **try not to panic** when the end is approaching. **Do not call 911**. If the paramedics are called, they may feel the need to resuscitate the patient and take him or her to the hospital. It is not unusual to become frightened, but call the hospice nurse rather than 911.

Often, hospice agencies offer **bereavement counseling/ classes** for individuals who have experienced recent loss. Some of these classes are open to people whose family members have not been a patient of the agency.

More information about Hospice can be obtained from the **Centers for Medicare and Medicaid Services CMS (www.cms.gov).**

Palliative care is a medical and nursing plan of care that focuses on providing **relief of symptoms** due to a disease, including pain. These are symptoms that not only can result from the illness, but also from the treatment of the disease, such as chemotherapy.

We discuss the use of palliative care at the end of one's life, but it is appropriate for all people who are dealing with an illness, especially a chronic illness. Just because someone is receiving palliative care, doesn't mean they cannot receive other lifesaving treatment. That occurs only if someone has chosen to receive hospice services.

Palliative care services include care not only from physicians and nurses, but also therapy, counseling, social services, pharmacy, and nutrition, just to name a few. Even massage therapy could play a part for some patient's treatment. The term **palliative means** to make less intense or less severe. That definition is a good description of the goal and scope of palliative care.

An **advantage** of receiving palliative care from a team of professionals with expertise in this area, is they have an understanding of effective measures to control symptoms. They are also able to assist the patient and family maneuver through the healthcare system.

Some of the main symptoms dealt with under palliative care include:

Pain is a major fear and concern for someone receiving palliative care. **Medication therapy** is the first line of pain control. The medical provider will begin pain control with the mildest medication regimen, that will control the pain and save the stronger drugs for later, especially if the condition involved is a chronic condition. Frequently, a **combination of medications** will be used to achieve satisfactory results with a minimal amount of side effects.

The medication regimen will be more effective, if the meds are taken before the pain becomes too severe.

The physician needs to **depend upon the patient's** input to assess the effectiveness of the pain control regimen. Only the patient can tell how much relief the medications provide. Healthcare professionals have developed a 10 point pain scale that helps the patients quantify their pain. (10 is the worst pain ever experienced by the patient, and 1 the least amount.) It helps the physician and nurses if the patient will keep a **record of pain rates** before and after pain medication administration and how often medication administration is necessary. Sharing this information with the healthcare personnel is helpful.

The **goal** is to avoid overmedicating in the beginning, which can lead to medication tolerance. This will improve the patient's ability to experience continued pain relief, as the disease progresses.

The physician will try to provide a form of medication that the **patient or caregiver can administer** themselves. The more control the patient has over when they receive their medications, the more they will be able to relax, leading to more effective pain control.

If the patient gets to the point where they need to receive medication by way of **injection,** including intravenous, the home-care or hospice nurse can come to the home to set up and supervise the IV therapy. They will also teach the patient or caregiver how to administer the medication.

Frequently, the physician can insert a permanent line into a vein to ease medication administration.

The **effects of pain medication** can be **enhanced** by use of relaxation and/or distraction therapies. Some of these **therapies include** a quiet, relaxed atmosphere using music, reduced lighting, massages, pleasant conversation, or an entertaining book. Other beneficial activities include TV or home movies, especially with humorous subjects.

Help patients find a comfortable position. Assist them when moving around so they avoid sudden moves that can cause extra pain. Sometimes, **relaxation exercises and/or guided imagery techniques** have been helpful in conjunction with the medication regime.

It helps to avoid stressful situations, cold damp environments, or becoming overtired. **Heat or ice** may be helpful in relieving pain. Avoid electric blankets and heating pads since they could cause burns.

Some common **side effects** experienced from pain medications are constipation, drowsiness, nausea, vomiting, and depressed respiration's.

Loss of appetite, Nausea & Vomiting, often, can be controlled with the administration of an anti-nausea medication. For the best results when nauseated, take the medication 30 minutes before meals. There can be many reasons why these symptoms are occurring. It can be due to the pain meds, the medical condition, treatment, or because of more than one of these factors.

Helpful measures, if nauseated, include:

- Take **small, frequent** meals.
- Avoid **spicy** foods.
- Increase calories with **high calorie, high protein foods** (ice cream, puddings).
- Sip **high protein** drinks.
- Serve foods **attractively**.
- Maintain a **quiet, sedate atmosphere** for meals.
- Avoid **noisy TV programs** at mealtime, especially news programs which can be upsetting.
- Avoid **controversial or upsetting** subjects during mealtime.
- Promote **pleasant conversations.**
- Avoid taking **large amounts of medications** just before meals, if not necessary.
- Avoid drinking **large amounts of liquids** with meals.
- Encourage client to **select foods** that sound good.
- Utilize **nutritionist** and/or **Speech-language** therapist, as needed.

Shortness of Breath is a common symptom in many medical conditions.

Suggested supportive measures for shortness of breath include:

- Keep **upper body elevated** to improve ease of breathing.
- **Pace activities** with rest periods.
- Keep primary **health provider informed** about respiratory status.
- Take related **medications,** as instructed.
- Avoid overuse of **pain medications**.
- Utilize **respiratory and/or oxygen therapy,** as needed.
- Encourage individual **not to smoke**.
- Do not allow **others to smoke** around the patient.
- Participate in **deep breathing and coughing** exercises, as instructed.

Fatigue is a frequent complaint of someone who is chronically ill or has a terminal illness. The level of fatigue will help dictate the level of assistance required.

Some suggestions for assistance with fatigue include:

- **Assist** with activities of daily living (bathing, walking).
- **Sit,** rather than stand, during activities whenever possible. (Example: Use a shower chair for bathing.)

- Provide **assistance** whenever moving about.
- Use **assistive devices,** such as a cane or walker.
- Make a point of **changing positions** and moving about on a regular basis.
- **Pace activities** with rest periods to conserve energy.
- Engage in short, frequent **periods of exercise**, depending upon the degree of fatigue (short walks or moving legs and arms while sitting or lying).
- If the patient is **too fatigued** to move extremities, the caregiver should assist.
- Wear sturdy, well-fitting **shoes** and clean **socks**.
- Physical and/or Occupational **Therapy** or a **nursing assistant** may be helpful.

Constipation is a common complaint of people experiencing chronic or terminal illness. There are 3 major factors that help promote regular bowel movements. Those factors are fluids, fiber, and activity.

Suggestions to help utilize these factors include:

- Drink 8-10 glasses of **fluid** per day.
- Drink **prune juice** at bedtime.
- Eat other **fibers,** such as green vegetables, every day.

- Promote **physical activity,** depending upon ability. (Examples: walking, leg & arm exercises, turning in bed with help.)
- Establish a **pattern** for bowel evacuation at the same time each day, after a meal.
- Administer a **suppository** 30 minutes before bowel evacuation time, as needed.
- Use a **stool softener**, as instructed by primary health provider.

Incontinence is the lack of or limited control of the bowel and/or bladder.

Suggested measures for incontinence are:

- **Do not** avoid **drinking fluids**. (This could lead to other problems such as bladder infections or dehydration.)
- Observe for the **frequency and time** of incontinence.
- Go to the bathroom about every two hours for urinary incontinence and after meals for bowel problems to promote an **elimination pattern.**
- A maneuver called **Crede'** is sometimes helpful to stimulate urination when on the toilet or bed pan.
- **Crede'** works by using firm downward strokes on the abdomen, from the umbilicus (belly button)

toward the bladder area, about 6-7 times and then exert firm pressure over the bladder to empty it.

- Waterproof **underwear** or **under pads** should be changed to keep the individual clean and dry.

Skin breakdown can be a problem when one becomes less mobile, the circulation becomes impaired, and the patient's nourishment decreases. Skin breakdown begins with a reddened area, but can progress to a deep pressure ulcer, if left unattended.

Measures to help prevent or minimize skin breakdown include:

- Keep skin **clean and dry**.
- **Bathe daily** (can be sponge baths).
- Pat on **lotion or moisturizer**.
- Avoid **scratching or rubbing** skin areas.
- Change **positions** frequently.
- **If bed bound**, do not let the individual lie in the same position longer than 2 hours.
- If possible, **walk** around every 1-2 hours.
- **Check bony/pressure areas** for redness, scratches, rashes, or other signs of skin breakdown.
- **Pressure or bony areas** include elbows, knees, ankles, back along the spine, and the coccyx area at the end of the spine.

- If **skin breakdown** is observed, notify doctor or nurse right away.
- Someone who is malnourished, can have skin breakdown just about anyplace on the body.
- **Cleanse** area thoroughly after toileting.
- If lack of bowel or bladder control, **change diapers** and/or **bed pads** whenever wet or soiled. (Exposure of **skin to urine and stool** will accelerate skin breakdown.)

Confusion and Restlessness can be factors for various reasons. It is expected if the individual has a form of dementia. But it can, also, occur when a person approaches death, due to reduced circulation to the brain and/or an increase of toxins in the body.

Measures to help promote orientation include:

- Watch for **signs of confusion.**
- **Use reminders** of time (clock) day, date (calendar), year, and location to reinforce orientation.
- **Reorient** to time, place, and date, when needed.
- Use reminders of people's **names and relationship.**
- Keep around **familiar objects** and keep patient in familiar **surroundings**.
- Keep the individual in a **safe environment.**
- Provide a means of **monitoring** the patient.

- If patient wanders, **provide safety** locks and alarms on doors.
- Wear medical ID at all times for people who wander.
- Provide a **signaling device** so patient can call for help, when needed.
- **Store medications** in a safe, secure place.
- Maintain a **regular routine** for care and events.
- Provide stimulating and divisional **activities.**
- **Correct** misunderstandings.
- Encourage **reminiscing**.
- Approach in **quiet, non-threatening** manner.
- **Avoid criticizing** patient.
- Allow patient time to accomplish **tasks**.
- Allow time to respond to **questions.**
- Provide a quiet, calm **environment**.
- Keep **physician** informed about mental status.

Grief is how one deals with the expectation of loss or actual loss of well-being. While dealing with the patient's grief is a priority, the rest of the family members and close friends, also, need to deal with their own grief. As a matter of fact, the better everyone is adjusting, the better they are going to be able to help the patient.

Measures to help promote coping with grief are:

- Spend time **sitting and visiting**.
- Allow **time for** patient to share feelings.
- Allow patient to talk about **feelings of death**.

- Assist with **problem solving** of concerns, related to impending disability and/or death.
- Allow patient to **determine the subject matter** of conversations.
- Sometimes **just sitting** with the individual, without talking, gives comfort.
- Encourage **reminiscing** with old photos and stories.
- Allow patient to have **control of decisions** about their care, as much as possible.
- **Include patient** in activities and decision making.
- Don't forget to include **young children** in visits and let them help with simple tasks.
- **Accept help** from spiritual advisor, social worker, or councilor, as appropriate.
- Utilize **cultural and spiritual rituals** that bring comfort for the individual.

Depression: Each individual is going to vary in the amount of depression they may experience when faced with a serious illness.

Some measures that may help the individual deal with depression are:

- Provide **support**.
- **Listen** to patient concerns.

- **Spend time** with them.
- **Notify** primary medical provider of mental status.
- Utilize professional **counseling/ social worker** or **spiritual** advisor.
- **Avoid stress** provoking situations.
- Encourage **relaxation and divisional** activities.

REMINDER: Refer to chapters in this book dealing with Safety Precautions and Common Medical Conditions for further information about needed care for specific conditions.

Approaching Death:

Signs that may be observed **as death approaches** include drowsiness, agitation, confusion, and increasing periods of unresponsiveness. There is a decreased need for food and fluids. There may be increased loss of bowel and bladder control, and increased labored, noisy, and irregular breathing. The skin becomes cooler, especially in the lower extremities, and discoloration may be observed in the legs.

Measures that may be helpful include:

- Plan **visits** for when person is alert.
- Provide a quiet, pleasant **atmosphere**.

- Continue to **talk** to the individual, even if he/she seems to be unconscious. (**Hearing** is believed to be the final sense to disappear.)
- Do not attempt to **restrain**.
- If restless, **protect** individual from injury.
- Be **calm** and **reassuring**.
- Provide **ice chips** and **sips of water**.
- Do not push **fluids,** if choking.
- Keep **lips and mouth** moist (i.e., lip balm, gel or spray mouth moisturizers).
- Keep individual **clean** and **comfortable**.
- **Reposition** every 2 hours for comfort and improved breathing.
- **Side lying position** may help promote breathing.
- **Elevate upper body** to ease respirations.
- Seek help from doctor or nurse to **manage increased saliva**.

Signs of death include: lack of pulse, breathing, and response. The jaw is relaxed, the pupils are dilated and fixed, and bladder contents are released.

There is no need to hurry in making calls and arrangements. If the individual has been under hospice care, most arrangements have already been made. Many families may want to take some time with the individual and/or pray or conduct other rituals.

Most states require that certain authorities be notified when someone dies at home. If the death is anticipated, the doctor or home care nurse will usually notify the authority beforehand so when the death occurs, a simple phone call is all that is necessary.

If under the management of a home care or hospice agency, the nurse can help make the necessary calls and prepare the individual's body for the funeral home.

CHAPTER XIX

PATIENT RIGHTS/ RESPONSIBILITIES

Healthcare providers must honor **the rights,** of their patients. They are also required to inform them of their rights, when admitted to their services. Unfortunately, when patients are first admitted to a healthcare service, they are given many pieces of paper. Since it tends to be a stressful time, these rights may get lost in the shuffle. Another issue that gets lost is the idea that, along with patient rights, there are patient responsibilities.

One of the major rights for a patient is the right of **confidentiality.** This has always been considered a right by the healthcare community, but it has also been a federally regulated right, enacted in 1996 under the **HIPAA** (Health Insurance Portability and Accountability Act). HIPAA forbids the sharing of **identifiable personal or medical information,** found in medical records. Healthcare employees **cannot** automatically share information with family or friends, except if the **patient gives permission** for that sharing. Usually that permission can be given verbally. Exceptions to that rule would be if the patient is a minor, or if the patient has an appointed representative.

Other patient rights and corresponding responsibilities include:

Rights	Responsibilities
Confidentiality:	Provide info about who may receive information.
Respect for patient and property:	Respect healthcare staff.
Individualized care:	Provide personal health information. Accept responsibilities for own health care. Assist in planning care.
Receive care without prejudice:	Accept care without prejudice
Refuse care:	Ask questions about purpose and benefits of care. Accept consequences of care refusal.
Information about care and resources:	Pay attention to information.

ELDER ABUSE/NEGLECT is a serious problem and may become more serious as our elder population continues to increase. Laws, regarding elder abuse, vary from state to state.

Elder abuse/neglect tends to be **underreported** for various reasons. **First**, if abuse takes place in the individual's home, the signs may go undetected. **Next,** the individuals may not be willing to ask for help because they are too embarrassed, especially if the abuser is a family member. The different types of abuse and neglect are **physical, emotional, sexual, and/or financial**.

Some signs of abuse/neglect are:

- Unexplained bruises, burns, broken bones.
- Suspicious scars.
- Witnessed verbal abuse.
- Display of fear by patient of another person.
- Intimidation or ridicule of elder.
- Habitual blaming.
- Unnecessary physical exposure.
- Missing money, valuables, or clothes.
- Unexplained money withdraws.
- Suspicious changes in will.
- Unpaid bills.
- Sudden changes in financial situation.
- Unusual weight loss and bed sores.
- Elder is unbathed.
- Unsanitary living conditions.
- Efforts to isolate elder.
- Unnecessary services or goods.

It is easy to understand why elder abuse, often, goes unreported. Many of these signs could be explained due to natural aging, leaving elders frail and more prone to injuries. Also relatives and friends find it hard to believe that someone they know would be abusive.

Many people hesitate reporting suspicions for fear they are mistaken. The state's **Adult Protective Services (APS)** are responsible to investigate the situation to make sure someone really is being abused, before any charges are made. Most states allow the reporter to remain **anonymous**. If the suspected abuse is taking place in a care facility, the long-term care **ombudsman** is a resource. All states have a **help line** that one can consult.

Some suggestions to prevent abuse include:

- **Check references** when hiring a caregiver or seeking out a care facility.
- **Provide respite** on a regular basis for the family caregiver, to prevent burnout.
- Utilize additional resources, such as **adult day care.**
- If possible, don't leave the full burden of care to **one person.**
- **Utilize support groups** for caregivers.
- Provide opportunities for **sleep.** (Sleep deprivation is common among caregivers.)
- **Monitor** the elder at different times of the day.
- **Ask** elder about bruises, etc.
- **Observe** elder/ caregiver interactions.
- Caregivers need to **ask for help** before they become too overwhelmed.
- Elders need to **avoid** becoming **isolated.**

- Elders and family should **keep informed** about potential **scams targeted toward the elderly**.
- **If** you are **experiencing abuse**, inform someone you trust, such as a family member, friend, or healthcare professional.

READING & SIGNING FORMS

One final issue: Over the years, I have been responsible for having many people (patients, family members, agents) **sign agreements, contracts, and permission forms**. It used to amaze me how readily people would sign those forms without reading them or asking questions.

It is especially important that patients understand what they are agreeing to when they sign surgical and procedural consent forms. They are supposed to be **informed consents,** in which the individual truly understands what is going to be done and its consequences.

It is also important that everything is **written accurately.** For example, if the procedure involves a particular side or extremity, you need to make sure the correct side is designated. It is errors like that which can lead to an even greater error, such as the amputation of the wrong extremity. If there is an error, a new form needs to be made.

It is the professional healthcare **provider, performing the procedure,** who is responsible to ensure the patient understands the procedure and its implications. This is true even if someone else is actually having you sign the document and witnesses your signature.

With the exception of an emergency, these documents should be **signed well ahead** of the surgery or procedure. This allows the individuals to **feel less pressure** when signing the document and helps them feel more free to **ask questions.**

Ideally, the form should be signed **before** the patient has any type of **sedation,** so they are clear-headed. It doesn't hurt to have your **spouse** or close **family member** present to help you ask questions.

The **main rules** one should follow when faced with having to **sign documents** include:

- Read the document thoroughly.
- Ask questions.
- Ensure accuracy.
- Do not rush.
- Make sure any modifications are added before signing.

CHAPTER XX

DEFINITIONS/RESOURCES

Activities of Daily Living: Activities that individuals use in their everyday life, such as bathing, dressing, eating, mobility and elimination, pp. 58, 132

Administration on Aging (www.aoa.gov): Federal services that provide funding to assist home and community based programs that help senior citizens and their caregivers remain in their own homes, for as long as possible pg. 22

Adult Protective Services (APS): State department that investigates reports of neglect, abuse, or exploitation of vulnerable adults, and reports findings to law enforcement. pp. 25, 246

Advanced Directives: Documents used to record individuals' wishes regarding medical and financial issues in the event they are no longer able to make decisions. pg. 213

Advocate: One who acts as a liaison between the elder and a health care provider or other type of agency. pg. 208

Affordable Care Act: Commonly known as Obamacare. Key features can be seen at (**www.healthcare.gov**/law/). pg. 35

Agent: One who represents an elder who is either mentally or physically incapable to handle their own affairs. pg. 214

Alanon (www.alanon.org): Organization that provides assistance and support for families and friends of addicted individuals. pg. 79

Alcoholic's Anonymous (www.aa.org): Provides assistance and support for alcoholics. pg. 79

Alzheimer's Association (www.alz.org): Organization that provides assistance and support for Alzheimer's disease patients and families pg. 136

American Academy of Orthopedic Surgeons (www.aaos.org): Web site that provides information for joint replacement surgery. **pg.** 116

American Cancer Society (www.cancer,org): Provides assistance and support for cancer patients and families. pg. 141

American Diabetes Association (www.diabetes.org): Provides support for diabetic patients and families. pg. 105

American Heart Association (www.heart.org): Provides support for cardiac patients and families. pg. 126

American Lung Association (www.lung.org): Supports patients and families with respiratory disorders. pg. 119

American Stroke Association (www.strokeassociation. org): Organization to assist stroke patients and their families.   pg. 134

Area Agencies on Aging (AAA): State agencies that administer the Area Agencies on Aging programs and services to assist senior citizens.   pg. 22

Arthritis: Inflammation of one or more joints of the body. Osteoarthritis and Rheumatoid are two types.   pg. 107

Arthritis Foundation (www.arthritis.org): Resource organization for patients and families dealing with arthritis.   pg. 116

Assisted Living Facilities: Provide apartments, rooms, or shared rooms and assistance with activities of daily living.   pg. 200

Board and Care Homes: Smaller facilities or residences that provide care to a limited number of residents.   pg. 200

Board Certification: Completion of requirements to practice medicine in certain specialty areas.   pg. 50

CaregiverStress.com: Resource for caregivers who care for family members at home.   pg. 183

Centers for Disease Control and Prevention (www.cdc. gov): Concerned with the nation's public health. Works with states to promote health, prevent and control infection, disease, and injuries, provide preparedness for environmental and health threats, and responds to health emergencies.   pg. 19

Centers for Medicare & Medicaid Services (www.cms.gov): Department of the Federal government which administers the Medicare and Medicaid services   pp. 10, 187

Cerebrovascular Accident (CVA): An interruption of blood flow to part of the brain, commonly known as a stroke.   pg. 130

Certified Nursing Assistant (CNA): Assists patients with activities of daily living and provide simple nursing care, such as taking vital signs. Must work under supervision of a nurse or physician. Education program includes at least 75 hours of classroom, lab practice and supervised clinical practice.   pg. 58

Chronic Obstructive Lung Disease (COLD) or Chronic Obstructive Pulmonary Disease (COPD): Disease characterized by obstruction of airflow in and out of lungs and loss of lung elasticity.   pg. 117

Congestive Heart Failure (CHF): A condition when the heart is unable to pump sufficient blood supply to meet the needs of the body.   pg. 126

Continuing Care Retirement Communities (CCRC): Communities consisting of apartments, condos, or houses that offer different levels of care, including SNF.   pg. 201

Co-payment: Amount paid by recipients for their share of the cost for medical services and supplies. Cost is usually a fixed amount.   pg. 29

Custodial Care: Non skilled personal care, such as assistance with eating, bathing, and ambulating (walking). These services are not paid for by Medicare.   pg. 34

Deductible: Annual amount paid by recipient for healthcare before insurance or Medicare begins payment.   pg. 32

Dementia: Loss of cognitive ability, which can include memory, problem solving, attention, and language.   pg. 134

Department of Agriculture (USDA), (www.usda.gov): My Pyramid (foodpyramid.com) My Plate (choosemyplate.gov) are nutritional services provided by this department.

pp. 74-105

Departments of Economic Security (DES): State agencies responsible for the safety and economic security of the citizens of that state. Services include adult and child protective services and independent living programs.

pg. 25

Department of Health and Human Services (HHS): Department of the Federal Government which administers the CDC, FDA, and CMS.   pg. 10

Departments of Health Services: State agencies for regulation and licensing of healthcare facilities, such as hospitals, nursing homes, and emergency medical services.   pg. 24

Diabetes Mellitus (DM): Chronic disease characterized by impaired sugar metabolism.   pg. 99

Do Not Intubate (DNI): Document indicating the individual does not want to be intubated (insertion of breathing tube) in the event they should stop breathing. pg, 215

Do Not Resuscitate (DNR): Document indicating the individual does not want to receive CPR in the event they should stop breathing or their heart stops. pg. 215

Durable Medical Power of Attorney: Document that names a proxy who will make health care decisions for an individual, if that person becomes unable to make decisions. pg. 214

Elder Abuse/Neglect: Involves physical, emotional, sexual, or financial mistreatment of an elder individual. pg. 244

Federal Employees Health Benefits Program (FEHBP): Provides health benefits for federal employees, including the US Congress and their dependents. pg. 20

General Practitioner: Physician who practices medicine in a general or family practice. pg. 47

Guardianship (Conservatorship, Fiduciary): Court appointed process to assign an individual to manage financial and/or personal affairs of an elder who has been deemed incapable of managing their own affairs. pg. 207

Gynecologist: Physician who specializes in women's general medical care for female conditions. pg. 48

Healthcare System: A multifaceted system of healthcare delivery from a variety of health professionals, that varies from State to State. pg. 1

Health Insurance Portability and Accountability Act (HIPAA): A confidentiality act that forbids the sharing of identifiable personal or medical information, found in medical records. pg. 243

Health Maintenance Organization (HMO): A managed care organization that provides healthcare services which focus on prevention of illness, for a fee. pg. 30.

Hospice Care: A full system of care for the terminally ill that involves alleviation of physical, emotional, and social symptoms. pg. 221

Hospitalist: Physician who specializes in the treatment of the hospitalized patient. pg. 49

Independent Practice Association (IPA): A group of independent practice physicians that contract with an HMO to provide medical services. pg. 31

Indian Health Services (www.ihs.gov): Provides health services to Native Americans, including Alaskan Natives. pg. 20

Internist: Physician who provides medical treatment for conditions that involve the body's internal systems. pg. 48

Leeuwen, Anne M. & Poelhuis-Leth, Debra J, Davis's Comprehensive Handbook of Laboratory and Diagnostic Tests with Nursing Implications, 3rd Ed, F.A. Davis, 2009.

Licensed Practical Nurse (LPN): Nurse who has completed at least a one year nursing program, successfully completed the State Board Examination for the LPN/LVN, and are licensed in the state in which they practice. Usually practices under the supervision of a registered nurse or physician. May also be titled Licensed Vocational Nurse (LVN)   pg. 50

Living Will: Document providing detailed instructions about medical care to be carried out if individuals are unable to voice their wishes.   pg. 213

Managed Care: Term used to describe programs designed to control the cost of healthcare services.   pg. 29

Medical Doctor (MD): Physician who is a graduate of a school of Medicine, completed an approved residency program, and successfully completed medical boards.
                                                                      pg. 46

Medicaid: Healthcare program provided for US citizens and legal aliens who live below a designated income level and have limited resources.   pg. 15

Medicare: Healthcare services provided for citizens who are 65 and older, disabled for at least 24-29 months, or have end stage renal disease.   pg. 10

Medicare Advantage: Federally approved programs that offer the same basic services as Medicare Parts A and B, and, also, may offer part D benefits. pg. 13

Medicare & You (www.docbig.com/Medicare/2013. Medicare.and.you): Booklet for Medicare recipients documenting Medicare benefits. pp. 10, 81

Medicare Coverage of Skilled Nursing Facility Care (www,cms.gov): Provides a SNF checklist to use when choosing a facility. pg. 192

Medigap: Secondary insurance, to be used in addition to Medicare. pg. 12

Monks, Karen, Home Health Nursing, Assessment and Care Planning, 4th Ed., Mosby, 2003.

Myocardial Infarction (MI): Heart Attack: interruption in blood flow to heart muscle, leading to muscle death. pg. 123

Narcotic's Anonymous (www.na.org): Support group for drug addicts. pg. 79

Nursing 2011 Drug Handbook, 31st Ed, Wolters Kluwer/ Lippincott Williams & Wilkins, 2011.

Nursing Home Compare (www.medicare.gov/NHcompare): Provides information about skilled nursing facilities. pg. 191

Nurse Practitioner: A registered nurse who has completed an advanced nursing education program, and is prepared to diagnose and treat common acute and chronic medical conditions.   pg. 46

Obstetrician: Physician who specializes in medical care focused on childbirth.   pg. 48

Occupational Therapist (OT): Therapist who has earned a master's degree from an accredited occupational therapy program, successfully completed the National Certification Examination of Occupational Therapy, and is licensed to practice. Provides therapy for clients, who experience mental, physical, developmental, and/or emotional disabilities, to achieve independence in their occupational, leisure, self care, domestic, and/or community activities.   pg. 53

Office of Personnel Management (OPM.): Federal Government office that administers the Federal Employees Health Benefits Program.   pg. 21

Ombudsman: Programs administrated by each state. Advocating services for residents in skilled nursing, assisted living, and other elder care facilities.   pp. 23, 191

Osteopathic Doctor (DO): Physician who is a graduate of a school of Osteopathy, completed an approved residency program, and successfully completes medical boards.   pg. 46

Palliative care: A multidiscipline approach to control physical, emotional, psychosocial, and spiritual symptoms of a disease.   pp. 143, 227

Pediatrician: Physician who specializes in the care of infants and children.   pg. 48

Pharmacist: Dispenses prescription medications. Graduates from a 4 year graduate program in pharmacy and successfully completes the North American Pharmacist Licensure Exam and pharmacy law exam.   pg. 54

Physical Therapist (PT): Therapists who have completed an accredited physical therapy program, successfully completed the national PT examination, and are licensed in the state in which they practice. Provides therapy for physical conditions related to injury, aging, disease, or environment.   pg. 52

Physician: A graduate of a school of medicine or school of osteopathy, completed an approved residency program, and successfully completed the medical boards.   pg. 46

Physician Assistant (PA): Licensed to provide medical treatment under the supervision of a physician. The scope of practice varies from state to state. PA education programs require that the candidates have some health care experience and the programs vary in length from a certificate to a master's degree.   pg. 56

Point of Service (POS): A type of managed care that combines characteristics of the HMO and PPO. pg. 33

Preferred Provider Organization (PPO): A managed care organization consisting of a group of physicians and/or other healthcare professionals that contract with a health insurance agency to provide healthcare at a reduced rate. pg. 32

Primary care Physician or Provider (PCP): The MD, DO or Nurse Practitioner, that you see first for your healthcare. Frequently, acts as a gatekeeper and provides referral to specialists, when needed. pg. 43

Psychiatrist: Physician who specializes in mental health treatment. pg. 48

Registered Nurse (RN): Nurses educated in an associate degree, bachelor of science degree, or diploma nursing program, successfully complete the NCLEX-RN test for licensure, and are licensed in the state in which they practice. pg. 51

Retirement Communities: Groups of homes, condos, or mobile homes, for people 55 years or older, that provide yard maintenance and recreation centers. pg. 199

Retirement Facilities: Provide individual apartments, along with meals, transportation, and housekeeping services. pg. 199

Respite Care: Housekeeping and nursing aide services provided to reduce stress for the caregiver. pg, 23

Skilled Nursing Facility (SNF): A nursing home that provides skilled nursing and/or rehabilitation services on a continuous, daily basis. pg. 185

Social Worker (BSW/MSW): Prepared in a bachelor's or master's degree social work program and may be either licensed or registered within the state they practice. The BSW usually practices under the supervision of an MSW, depending upon the practice setting. pg. 55

Specialty Healthcare Insurances: Types of insurance policies that pay for treatment for specific conditions, such as cancer, or circumstances, such as long term care. pg. 33

Speech-Language Pathologist (SLP): Therapist who has earned a master's degree in speech pathology, completed 375 hours of supervised clinical experience, passed the National Speech-Language Pathology examination, and completed at least 9 months post graduate experience. The SLP is licensed in the state of practice. Provides therapy for clients experiencing issues related to speech, language, and/or communication. pg. 54

State Health Insurance Assistance Programs (SHIP): Provides counseling to help Medicare beneficiaries and their families make informed decisions about Medicare and supplemental insurance coverage. pg. 27

Surgeon: Physician who specializes in the treatment of injuries, disease, and deformities through the use of surgery.   pg. 48

Therapy Aide: Usually trained on the job to provide clerical assistance and help ready the treatment area and equipment for the therapist.   pg. 57

Therapy Assistant: Prepared to assist with the implementation of the therapy care plan under the supervision of the therapist. Educational preparation involves completion of a minimum of an associate degree in the discipline in which they are working. Regulation varies from state to state which may require a license, certification, or registration. pg.57

Third Party Payers: Establishments (government and private) which finance healthcare for the patient . pg. 7

Transient Ischemic Attack (TIA): An episode of temporary symptoms of a stroke.   pg. 131

Veterans Affairs (www.va.gov): Provides health care services for veterans who have been discharged from active military service, as long as the discharge was not dishonorable.   pg. 21

ABOUT THE AUTHOR

Karen McGough Monks is married to Patrick, has two adult children, and two grandchildren. She resides in Yuma, Arizona.

The author is a retired nurse of 50 years. She graduated from a diploma nursing program in 1956, earned a bachelor's degree in nursing at Marquette University in Milwaukee, Wisconsin in 1965, and earned a master's degree in nursing at the University of Texas Medical Branch in 1984.

Her work experience included positions in medical centers and an extended care facility as a staff nurse, head nurse, and house supervisor.

When she married Patrick, they moved to Arizona, where she took a position in the local community hospital. In the early 1970s, she took a nursing instructor position in an associate degree nursing program, at a community college. She spent 23 years with the nursing program, including 8 years as director of the program.

During the time spent with the nursing program, the author, also, was a member of the local hospital's board of directors for 12 years, an accreditation visitor for associate degree nursing programs, and a member of the National League for Nursing board of review, which evaluates nursing programs. Additionally, she worked part-time as a home-care nurse.

In 1995, Karen retired from the nursing program and took a position as an educator for a home care agency. She retired at the age of 70. During the early 2000s, she published two handbooks for home care professionals.

Made in the USA
Columbia, SC
05 July 2025

60351981R00154